# IMMUNE POWER

## DR. I. WILLIAM LANE
## SUSAN BAXTER

Foreword by
Dr. Mamdooh Ghoneum

AVERY PUBLISHING GROUP
Garden City Park • New York

The advice in this book is based on the training of, experiences of, and pool of information available to the authors. Mention of any research organization or individual researcher should in no way be construed as an endorsement of this book or of any techniques therein. Because each person and situation are unique, the editor and the publisher urge the reader to check with a qualified health professional when there is any question regarding the presence or treatment of any abnormal health condition. The publisher does not advocate the use of any particular treatment, but believes that the information in this book should be available to the public.

Because there is always some risk involved, the author and publisher are not responsible for any adverse effects or consequences resulting from the use of any of the preparations or procedures described in this book. Please do not use this book if you are unwilling to assume the risk. For personalized advice, please consult a physician or other qualified health professional. It is a sign of wisdom, not cowardice, to seek a second or third opinion.

Cover Design: Eric Macaluso
Cover Photo: PhotoDisc
Typesetter: Richard Morrock
Editor: Claudette Upton

**Avery Publishing Group**
120 Old Broadway
Garden City Park, NY 11040
1–800–548–5757
www.averypublishing.com

The illustration on page 36 (right) and the photos on page 142 and 143 were provided courtesy of Dr. Mamdooh Ghoneum.

The photo on page 36 (left) was provided courtesy of the Cancer Research Institute of West Tennessee.

**Library of Congress Cataloging-in-Publication Data**
Lane, I. William
    Immune power: how to use your immune system to fight disease—
from cancer to AIDS / I. William Lane, Susan Baxter.
    p. cm.
    Includes bibliographical references and index.
    ISBN 0-89529-934-8
    1. Natural immunity. 2. Immune system. 3. Biological response
modifiers. I. Baxter, Susan. II. Title.
    QR185.2.L36  1999
    616.07'9—dc21                                                99-16122
                                                                          CIP
                                                                          r99

Copyright © 1999 by I. William Lane

Printed in the United States of America

10 9 8 7 6 5 4 3 2 1

# Contents

## Part Four  Cooperating With the Immune System

*In memory of our friend
Jill Leach.*

# Foreword

Starting with my early education in Egypt, I have been fascinated by the workings of the immune system. Later, during my four years of doctoral work in Japan, followed by my teaching and research career in California, immunology became my life.

Many scientists work for years looking for something that will make a contribution to society. I had been conducting research on a variety of natural substances said to have immune-boosting properties when one product distinctly attracted my attention. It was a rice bran product called MGN-3—a product that has since consumed nearly all my time and effort. After promising preliminary studies, my research team of scientists and medical doctors found dramatic clinical implications for this project among cancer patients. Every new study reveals more about its ability and potential for helping individuals with serious health conditions.

I have published many of my findings, but have found to my dismay that my papers and work are overlooked by many in the scientific community. This is often the case with natural therapies. In 1996, a breast cancer patient who had exhausted all the possibilities offered by conventional medicine tried my therapy. She is now cancer free. In 1998, this patient introduced me and my work to Dr. I. William Lane, who immediately saw the same significant potential that I had recognized. Together we have been publicizing—both to the lay public and to those professionals who will listen—the remarkable capability of MGN-3, a simple but complex product.

This book is about the workings of the immune system, and

specifically about the workings of natural killer cells (NK cells), which are considered to be the body's first line of defense against cancer and viral infections. You will see how often conventional drugs work against rather than with the immune system that protects us. Many medical doctors trained in Western drug-oriented medicine are now discovering the possibilities and functions of the immune system. The alternative medical community must now begin to approach the conventional medical community using a language that is understandable to them—that is, the results of clinical studies that show scientifically proven methods of healing.

It is my hope that *Immune Power* will alert tens of thousands of cancer, hepatitis, and HIV patients—as well as individuals suffering from other serious illnesses—to proven natural therapies. Hopefully, in the future, prevention rather than treatment will get more attention. I anticipate that MGN-3 will be a major force in this movement.

Mamdooh Ghoneum, Ph.D.
Chief of Research
Drew University of Medicine and Science

# Preface

*"Medicine sometimes snatches away health, sometimes gives it."*
—Ovid (43 BC–c. AD 17), Roman poet

When healthy people get sick, usually their first impulse is to race over to the doctor's office or the emergency ward to get whatever it is "fixed." Sometimes they're lucky, and the doctors can find the root cause of their illness—remove an inflamed appendix, give antibiotics for a bacterial infection, set a broken bone. Unfortunately, there's also an alarmingly high number of disabling conditions—chronic diseases, most cancers, syndromes, and other instances of poor health—where traditional Western medicine is helpless. There is no root cause, no definite "problem" that surgery can eradicate or drugs can cure. And even though modern medical research has brought enormous advances in our understanding of health and disease, we still know far less about the origin and perpetuation of disease than is popularly thought.

In my view, a large part of the problem has to do with the theoretical framework that modern Western medicine has taken on, namely that of ignoring the workings of the body itself. It's like that old medical joke: The operation was a great success; it's a pity the patient had to die.

Many people know my work on shark cartilage and the years I've spent researching it and writing and speaking about it. What fewer people know is that—perhaps because of my background in science, coupled with a tendency to stick my neck out for the things I believe in—I've also delved into areas other than shark cartilage, though always related to health. Sometimes, the researcher or scientist came to me; at other times it was their patients, or other people who knew of their work, who contacted me and said, "Look, Dr. Lane, this is an extraordinary discovery and you've got to help Dr. X tell people about it."

That's pretty much what happened with MGN-3 (Arabin-oxylan Compound) and Mamdooh Ghoneum, Ph.D., a respected California immunologist who is chief of research in the Department of Otolaryngology (the medical specialty that's involved with the ear, nose, and throat) at Drew University of Medicine and Science, affiliated with UCLA. One of Dr. Ghoneum's clinical subjects, a woman who had had cancer, got in touch with me to tell me about MGN-3, a natural, nontoxic, patented substance originating in Japan. It's made from rice bran treated with the enzymes of shiitake mushrooms and consists mostly of hemicellulose, a kind of dietary fiber.

Dr. Ghoneum encountered MGN-3 in 1991 and spent the next eight years researching it, painstakingly starting with laboratory rats, then working up to studies using human blood, and finally to human subjects. In the process, he found that MGN-3 had an extraordinary effect on the immune system, in particular in strengthening the natural killer (NK) cells that are our bodies' primary natural defense against tumors and against viral diseases.

The immune system is probably one of the least-known of our bodily functions. Yet it is probably *the* most important one. If our immune system doesn't work, then we're dead. This complicated array of B cells, T cells, NK cells, and macrophages, among other cells—as you'll see in this book—are our bodies' built-in defense against disease, and against invasion from bacteria, viruses, and other microorganisms. Thus, its seamless functioning is the single most powerful force we have to keep us healthy. But until AIDS showed us the important role the immune system plays in our bodies, there was hardly any research going on in this subject. Nobody really believed that the immune system mattered. Except people like Dr. Ghoneum.

The more information that was accumulated on MGN-3, the more amazing it was. At first, Dr. Ghoneum had thought merely that MGN-3 would work with cancers that were in the bloodstream or bone marrow, like leukemia or multiple myeloma. But as he did more studies, he found that it was also effective for solid tumors like those that occur in the breasts, ovaries, and prostate. MGN-3 even had properties that controlled AIDS. Now it turns out that it may also help combat hepatitis, chronic fatigue, and a host of other conditions we still haven't fully studied. Unfortunately, as the woman who contacted me realized, outside of Japan, MGN-3 was unknown to the people who really needed it: people with cancer who had undergone traditional treatments like chemotherapy and radiation and whose immune systems (and NK cells in particular) were depleted, tired, and just too weak to fight off the remaining or returning cancer; people with AIDS, with only a short while to live; sick people who were trying to get better; people in need of hope and health; people that the medical establishment too often ignores. So that's where I came in.

This book came about because of MGN-3, Dr. Ghoneum, and my involvement with this substance when I realized just how amazing it really is. But it's not possible to talk about an immunotherapeutic agent and explain how it works without also explaining the complexities of the immune system. So this book begins with a description of your immune system, how it works, and how its workings were discovered late in the nineteenth century. You'll learn about what happens when you get something as simple as a cold or as complex as an autoimmune disorder. We cover all the immunological bases—from allergies to AIDS, stress to cancer. Then we tell you how this knowledge can assist you to use your own body's power, your own immune system's strengths, to stay healthy and to combat disease.

I'm really excited about MGN-3 and its potential to help people with cancer, AIDS, hepatitis, and a lot of other things. I think that once you understand immunity and how you can make it work for you—not against you, as so many medical treatments end up doing—you will be excited too. Immunity is strength. Knowledge is power. And the two of these together are truly a force to be reckoned with.

I. William Lane, Ph.D.
Short Hills, New Jersey
and Daytona Beach, Florida

# Introduction

*"To believe in medicine would be the height of folly, if not to believe in it were not a greater folly still."*
—Marcel Proust (1871–1922), French writer

This is a book about the immune system and about MGN-3, a remarkable dietary supplement that modulates the immune system and increases the activity of a certain kind of white blood cell known as natural killer (NK) cells. These cells are antiviral and antitumor, and their strong and active presence is often a sign of robust good health and the ability to fend off disease. Yet much of modern life—from stress to pollution—has an adverse effect on these and other immune cells.

When we first discussed the writing of this book, we agreed that this was an important topic that people deserved to hear about. But it wasn't possible to write just about NK cells or immune modulation without putting it in the larger context of the immune system. After all, a balanced, well-functioning immune system is essential to good health. Yet most of us (including us, at the time!) know very little about it. There aren't a lot of books or articles on the subject, and what little there is tends to be academic, technical, and difficult to read. We wanted to change that.

When you write about medicine, it's sometimes difficult not to get downright cynical about a lot of medical news. Every day, we hear the latest "news" on how they've found a cure, or at least the latest treatment, for everything from athlete's foot to AIDS—no matter that some of this late-breaking information contradicts yesterday's news. But if you look at the big picture and talk to real people—to patients—you start to see the cracks. Most medical strategies leave a lot to be desired when it comes to healing the whole person. More often than not, their impact on an individual's quality of life is quite negative.

Yes, we've come a long way in controlling disease, but too many people who end up mired in the medical system end up stressed, scared, and abandoned. The mere fact that assisted suicide is even a topic of discussion demonstrates that.

This book covers the immune system for the average person. We have tried to make it as readable as possible, using plenty of examples, analogies, and word "pictures." It is complicated in places—but so is the immune system. We begin with a description of the basics of immunity and how it works, covering all the bases from cellular dynamics to the history of the smallpox vaccine. Later, we move on to things that can go wrong with the immune system, from allergies to asthma to autoimmune disorders and AIDS. Then, we cover solutions—what you can do to help your immune system along. Immune power, in other words.

A healthy immune system wards off disease, even cancer. It is self-regulating and knows when to get involved and when to stay in the background. In the end, it's all that stands between us and a hostile world.

Susan Baxter

# Part One

---

# Immune
# System Basics

# Chapter 1

# The Defining Nature of Immunity

*"I think, therefore I am."*
—René Descartes (1596–1650), French philosopher
and mathematician

*"I think I think; therefore, I think I am."*
—Ambrose Bierce (1842?–1914), U.S. satiric writer

How do you know you're you? In other words, how do you *know* you exist? Because you think? Because you feel? Because you take up space? At first glance, the question may seem silly. Of course you know you exist. Even as a child you knew that you were unique; that you were different from everybody else; that you were "you."

Psychologically, personally, it's not that difficult to define the self. We all know intuitively that it is our thoughts, feelings, memories, emotions, beliefs, morals, and actions that add up to a singular total: a unique sum of all our intellectual, behavioral, and social parts that interact with the world. But what makes us *physiologically* unique? What keeps you physically intact, distinct from other people, and makes *you* a biological entity separate from me and everybody else?

In a word: immunity. Your immune system.

From the outer layer of your skin, which acts as a physical barrier between you and the rest of the world, all the way inside to your heart, lungs, liver, and other internal organs, it's your immune system that determines who you are, keeps you intact, and maintains your boundaries. As an entity—a self-contained being—you would not exist without your immune system; like water, which can be poured from one glass to another, you would be fluid. Anything, from a microbe to a bacterium to any other foreign body, could simply attach itself to you at any time and become "part" of you. Like a vast, uncharted territory through which anyone can pass without passport or border patrols, you would be penetrable, open, and without boundaries. No physical limit would determine you, your "self." Your organs would be interchangeable with anyone else's; your heart or kidney or brain could function just as easily in another body as in your own. Organ transplants would be a breeze—no messing around with anti-rejection drugs and blood typing and size—but then, who'd need them?

## IMMUNE MISCONCEPTIONS

Most of us vaguely know that our immune system is there to protect us and keep us safe from "germs" and other foreign "invaders." We have all had vaccines and understand that somehow, by giving us a watered-down version of potentially deadly diseases, they protect us from the real thing. We realize that the sore throat, cough, and aches and pains of a cold are our bodies' defenses, set in motion by our immune system fighting the virus. AIDS has brought discussions about the immune system to the front pages, and on TV and the radio we hear references to T cells and B cells and so on. But, by and large, the immune system is just another one of those mysterious inner workings that we take for granted, like digestion or breathing or heartbeat. It's only an issue when it doesn't work, or when there's something seriously wrong.

This attitude about the immune system has been largely shared by scientists. Although knowledge of how immune processes work increased dramatically from the nineteenth century onward—

thanks primarily to advances in the study of bacteria, or *bacteriology*—even the notion of an immune *system* did not develop until 1978. For years, what was known about immune functions was assumed to be the result of various separate units functioning independently, in isolation from one another. The idea that these worked in concert, like an orchestra playing a symphony, seemed too outrageous to believe. But gradually (mainly because of the growing understanding of AIDS), the immune system began to be seen as an integrated, coordinated, and organized whole: a complex array of cell functions that not only keep us "safe" from invading microorganisms but are a vital link to other physiological functions.[1]

## TO PROTECT AND DEFEND

Infinitely complex, "the carefully orchestrated cellular immune system operates physiologically as the major impediment to infections and consequently has a major survival value for the species," remarks an immunology textbook.[2] Like the finest of sharpshooters, it is able to take perfect aim at dangerous invaders. Superbly regulated, the immune system usually displays an unerring instinct to fend off the microorganisms that cause disease, in order to protect itself and, by extension, the host organism—you. Its most basic function, then, is to recognize what is *autologous*, self (you), and what is foreign, or not-self.

This simple "okay/not-okay" distinction is essential, since any physiological system that is armed to destroy must be able to distinguish between the materials of its own body and those that are not of its body. In some ways, the immune system is comparable to an army, equipped to kill, which must be able to know who's on their side and who's the enemy; they must be able to recognize uniforms, passwords, flags, and all the other defining insignia. This is not as easy as it sounds, because all living creatures are built from the same building blocks of nature—proteins, amino acids, DNA, and so forth (see the inset "Self and Not-Self: In the Beginning" on page 8).

# Self and Not-Self: In the Beginning

*The fact that the natural building blocks that make up all organisms are so similar—whether the organism is an amoeba or an armadillo, a human or a horse—has led some scientists to speculate that the immune system might long ago have been some kind of organism itself. According to the theory, this "being" attempted to find a foothold for itself within a safer, smaller environment, since the world was undoubtedly a very threatening place millions of years ago. This provocative idea suggests that the first immune cells might have been amoeba-like creatures—perhaps even parasites—wandering about in the early ocean, which then "invaded" early animals whose bodies were safer than the ocean itself. This gave the cells a site in which they could more easily survive: a place to call home. Or, perhaps, these early microscopic invaders were actually invited in or even "conscripted" by ancient organisms because of their ability to repel or destroy other tiny invaders that posed a threat.[1]*

*The relationship would have been of mutual benefit: both organism and host would have increased their odds of survival and of reproducing their own genetic material through the long and exhaustive evolutionary process. No doubt, as the ancient creatures began to leave the oceans, the need to "police" the internal environment, to distinguish between self and not-self, became a more pressing matter than it had been when all life oozed around in the "primordial soup." Backup for this seemingly bizarre theory is actually not hard to find, given that so many human immune reactions, at their most basic and nonspecific, so closely resemble those of invertebrates, even sponges and starfish.*

*Embryologist Edward Zwilling[2] performed an elegant experiment on one of the most primitive sea creatures around: sponges. These sea organisms have primitive nervous systems and no movement of body parts. Yet even these organisms can distinguish between one another on a cellular level, can "know" what consti-*

> *tutes self as opposed to not-self. Zwilling put two species of sponge into a blender and mixed them all up so that all the cells of one sponge mingled completely with those of the other. But within moments of being left alone, individual cells from the two sponges swiftly and unerringly resegregated into the two original sponges (though slightly rearranged). The process, apparently, resembled the kind of trick we see on television when a broken vase or smashed object swooshes back into its original shape through the magic of reverse-time photography—except that with the sponges, it was no trick. Their cellular individuation and reversal back into their original "selves" really happened.*

## AN ADAPTABLE DEFENSE SYSTEM

Even though, at its most basic level, the immune system does protect or defend the integrity of the biological self, this complicated array of cellular activity is more than simply defensive. True, it does battle microorganisms, similar to the way armies and navies protect a nation from a foreign threat; but immunity is more elaborate than that. Like human society, it's bewilderingly multi-layered, a busy network that somehow takes stock of all the normal tissues in our bodies, retains a memory of past encounters with foreign microorganisms, and then adjusts itself as it goes along.[3] Daily, it sifts through a gigantic amount of information and misinformation, and, like the most complicated computer systems, decides what to react to and what to ignore or adapt to. Its most obvious function is indeed defensive, which we've known since the nineteenth century; but in its connections and interconnections it is considerably more sophisticated than previously believed. It is fluid and dynamic, adaptive and street-smart, much more like a savvy con artist than like the impeccably tailored Prussian general it was seen as twenty or thirty years ago.

The immune system's limits, furthermore, are not as definite as we used to think. The world—the environment we live in—is a rapidly changing place, and the immune system has to be similarly changeable. Much in the way that the French realized during World War II that their "line in the sand," the Maginot Line, was hopelessly inadequate when it came to German air attacks, we've now come to realize that our rather old-fashioned notions about the immune system as an impenetrable fortress, shielding us against all outside threats ranging from bacteria to fungi, is similarly outdated. In any event, it would be both futile and counterproductive for the immune system to attempt to repel *every* microbe and parasite that attempted entry. Many of these, as it happens, are helpful and necessary for ordinary healthy human functioning.

Bacteria in the intestinal tract, for instance, help us digest food and keep the area clean of other harmful invaders. To get rid of *all* foreign material leads to problems, as anyone who's taken antibiotics and developed stomach problems can attest. It would be neither sensible nor protective for our immune systems to keep us perfectly "sterile" all the time; there are simply too many microorganisms out there.

Then there are times when the immune system gets it wrong. Allergies, asthma, autoimmune disorders: these are all cases where the immune system gets its wires crossed. The responsiveness of the immune system can translate into trouble. Today, we're also seeing increasing numbers of people whose immune systems, for various reasons, are weak, faulty, or inadequate.

## "BUBBLE BOY"

The most dramatic example of immune inadequacy in recent years was the boy whose life was lived out in the media. David, better known as the "Bubble Boy" (his last name was never revealed out of respect for his family's privacy), was born in Houston, Texas, on September 21, 1971, with a rare genetic defect known as severe combined immune deficiency (SCID). SCID strikes roughly one of every 150,000 babies born in the United States. Babies born with this condition have, in essence, no functional immune system. In other words, they can't fend off viruses or bacteria or other disease-producing organisms. David's parents and doctors hoped that by keeping David in his "bubble," a totally sterile environment free of the bacteria, fungi, and viruses that could so easily kill him, he would eventually develop a fully mature immune system (which has been known to happen, apparently). In David's case it never did.

For twelve years, David lived in his bubble, though he was briefly outfitted with a special suit, a bit like the ones astronauts wear, so he could venture outside. Unfortunately, getting him in and out of the gear proved to be far too difficult, and he soon outgrew it anyway. Although highly intelligent and "healthy" according to his medical records, David never touched another human being or led a life that could be considered in any way normal. Eventually, at his own urging, David underwent an experimental procedure when he was twelve years old. His sister, Katherine, not a perfect match but the closest they could find, donated bone marrow that was pre-treated with an experimental monoclonal antibody treatment. The bone marrow was then transplanted into David. The hope was that Katherine's bone marrow would supply David with the immune system he lacked. It didn't. Tragically, there were traces of Epstein-Barr virus (EBV) in his sister's bone marrow (even though she'd never developed any symptoms from it), and David got terribly ill. The autopsy found that the antigens present in Katherine's bone marrow were enough for David's immune system to create tumors, tumors made up of his own B cells. This shows just how easily a common virus like EBV can, without appropriate immune intervention, kill. David died on February 22, 1984, a monument to something—what, exactly, we don't know.

David's story is a graphic and unhappy demonstration of how essential our immune system is to our survival and the extent to which it is specific to each person alone. As flawed as his immune system was, David still managed to survive, to live, in the bubble, which was an environment tailored to his needs. But once his sister's bone marrow, with its own antibodies, was transplanted into him, even though their genes were so similar, his body rebelled. By the same token, each and every one of us survives because our immune systems make it possible for our internal environment to stay uniquely ours. By recognizing foreign particles (at a cellular level) and either co-opting them into our selves or destroying them, our immune system ensures that we survive, genetically and biologically intact, as unique beings.

## TWENTIETH-CENTURY DISEASES?

David's is not the only immune-system story we've seen or heard from the media. Regularly, we hear about children needing transplants or complicated medical procedures to correct faulty hearts or kidneys or other life-threatening conditions. Less dramatic, but increasing all the time, are allergies and asthma—essentially a case of the immune system's misreading and reacting against what should be a harmless environmental stimulus, like pollen or a bee sting. Then there are those whose immune systems turn on them with diabetes, multiple sclerosis, lupus, rheumatoid arthritis, and other autoimmune diseases that have crippling and sometimes fatal consequences. To what extent these immune-system aberrations are a modern phenomenon—a result of the toxins and other pollutants that we are increasingly exposed to—is a matter of heated debate.

Some scientists believe that prior to the eighteenth century, many autoimmune diseases did not exist. For instance, there is no convincing medical description of rheumatoid arthritis (RA)—a disease of the immune system—in European medical literature before the nineteenth century, though some 3,000- to 5,000-year-old North American skeletons have recently been found to have bone erosions compatible with RA. There is some speculation that RA originated in the New World, perhaps as a result of some type of allergen or microorganism.[4] Osteoarthritis, in contrast, which is a result of wear and tear, has been observed in skeletal remains of Neanderthal man, dating back over 40,000 years.

Today there are even people diagnosed with allergies (or possibly sensitivities) to *everything*, who, in order to survive, have gone to live in the desert in homes made entirely of natural materials. It is still not known whether this "twentieth-century disease" is actually an immune-mediated reaction, a hypersensitivity to the many chemicals and additives in our environment, a psychiatric disorder, or some yet-to-be-discovered disease, but what is not in question is that these people are genuinely suffering. And in both developing and developed nations, chemicals, pollutants, and other stresses—both physiological and psychological—are having an impact. So many people are dying of cancer and AIDS that these diseases have been referred to as epidemics of our times.

## PLAGUES AND EPIDEMICS

A disease that seems to be defeating our attempts at control or cure is often referred to as an *epidemic.* We talk about an epidemic of breast cancer, or the AIDS epidemic. Historically, epidemics and plagues have often given us new ideas about immunity. For centuries it was known, for example, that someone who had had certain diseases and survived would not catch the same diseases again. The Greek historian Thucydides wrote that when the plague raged through Athens during the second year of the Peloponnesian War (around 500 BC), many more of the sick would have died without the care and nursing of those who'd *recovered* from the plague. So even 2,500 years ago, somebody did notice that nobody caught the plague a second time.

Formerly, the term "plague" was used to describe any epidemic causing great mortality, but now it refers to a specific infectious disease caused by the bacillus *Pasteurella pestis.* There are three forms of plague: *bubonic,* characterized by "buboes" or swelling of the lymph nodes, which is not uncommon in the presence of an infection; *pneumonic,* which involves the lungs; and *septicemic,* which invades the bloodstream and is so rapidly fatal that the other two forms have no time to develop symptoms. Primarily a disease of rats and other rodents, and spread by the rat flea, plague spreads to humans through infected animals or flea bites—which, in the slums of olden times, was common enough. Even today, cities harbor plenty of rats, usually around garbage bins and other sites where there is spoiling food—and the plague has still not been eradicated.

During the fourteenth century, when the plague (then called the Black Death) spread across Europe, an estimated 25 million people—a quarter of the population of Europe—died of either bubonic or pneumonic plague. The Great Plague of London in 1664–1665 resulted in 70,000 deaths (out of a total population of 460,000). "Thence I walked to the Tower; but Lord! how empty the streets are and how melancholy, so many poor sick people in the streets full of sores," the famous British diarist Samuel Pepys wrote on September 16, 1665. "[In] Westminster, there is never a physician and but one apothecary [pharmacist] left, all being dead." Pepys faithfully recorded numbers: "In the City died this week 7496 and of them 6102 of the plague. But it is feared that the true number of the dead this week is near 10,000—partly from the poor that cannot be taken notice of through the greatness of the number, and partly from the Quakers and others that will not have any bell ring for them" (August 31, 1665). Thankfully, Pepys writes, by November of that year the dead were down to 1,300 a week, "for which the Lord be praised."

Pepys's aunt died of the plague, as did some other members of the middle and upper classes, but the majority of plague victims were poor, malnourished, and living in unsanitary conditions, and therefore had weakened immune systems. We are not immune to "plagues" or epidemics today, particularly in those parts of the world where there is extreme poverty. Between 1969 and 1993, 36,643 cases of the plague in Africa, Asia, North America, and South America were reported to the World Health Organization (WHO).[5]

Other epidemics rage today that are just as virulent—some better known than others. Tuberculosis (TB) still kills more youth and adults each year than any other infectious disease.[6] The World Health Organization estimates that unless treatments improve, 70 million people will die of TB in the next twenty years.

But TB is old news; the worst epidemic today is the one that ravages the immune system itself. Human immunodeficiency virus, or HIV, the virus that most scientists believe precedes AIDS, attacks the immune system, leaving it powerless against infection and disease. By 1995 the death toll from AIDS had surpassed half a million in the United States, and an estimated 6 million people have died of AIDS worldwide to date,[7] 2.3 million in 1997 alone.[8] It is not actually AIDS, however, that kills these people but other, "opportunistic" infections that would be controlled or kept in check by a healthy immune system. Like David, the Bubble Boy, AIDS is a sharp reminder to us that the immune system plays a vital role in health—and AIDS has been largely responsible for the renewed interest in immunology in the past decade or so.

## THE POWER OF KNOWLEDGE

Recent years have seen enormous breakthroughs in the science of immunology, particularly with respect to its component parts—though there is still much that we don't know about why and how the immune system functions as it does. There's increasing evidence, however, that this growing field of study is going to hold many of the keys to disease and, by extension, to health. It is, after all, our immune system that keeps us healthy and prevents disease from taking hold time and time again. But what makes one person become ill with cancer and another not? What makes one person catch the cold that's going around and another not? Undoubtedly the answer has to do with the subtle interplay of our genes, our environment, and even our personalities and our individual ability to deal with stress. But most important is how these unique characteristics affect the workings of the immune system itself—and therefore each person's ability to fend off disease.

One of the major causes of the devastation of North American indigenous populations 500 years ago was infectious diseases, brought by European settlers into settlements populated by Native Americans whose immune systems had never been exposed to common European *pathogens* (causes of disease, such as viruses and bacteria).[9] Never having been exposed to the childhood diseases considered to be commonplace in Europe, like measles and mumps—not to mention smallpox—the native people became sick, and great numbers of them died. They would have been particularly vulnerable in years when the winter had been unusually cold or the harvest poor, because malnutrition and general ill health would have weakened their immune systems.

Today, we know a great deal about the disease process and about how the body works. But at least with respect to the immune system, that knowledge is largely reductionist[10] and piecemeal. The next major hurdle facing us is to understand immunity more holistically and systematically, and to work through testable theories to find clinical solutions. But to do that, we need to understand disease better. As the Greek essayist and biographer Plutarch (AD 46–120) said nearly 2,000 years ago, "Medicine, to produce health, has to examine disease." For, in the long run, we can't understand what it means to be well without knowing what can go wrong—and how. Fundamentally, what this means is that we need a basic understanding of the immune system and how it works. In the next few chapters, we will explore the various levels of immunity and immune-system response.

# Chapter 2

# Generalized Defenses

*"The diseases which destroy a man are no less natural than the instincts which preserve him."*
—George Santayana (1863–1952), Spanish-born U.S. philosopher, poet, and critic

Imagine that you're sitting somewhere, calmly reading a book, when suddenly someone spills a glass of milk over you. But thanks to that marvelous "packaging," skin, your outermost most basic barrier, this mishap is only a slight nuisance, not a major threat (unless you happen to be wearing a black suit). Skin—particularly the tough outer layer—ensures that external particles, from dust mites to crumbs, don't penetrate into you. This outer layer alone is enough to protect us from many different types of infection—which explains why a cut or scrape, where the skin is actually broken, can become infected so easily. It's like a broken fence post that lets in any stray animals that want to wander in. In addition to simply existing as a protective barrier, skin secretes oily substances that are themselves able to kill some bacteria, and an enzyme, also present in tears, that attacks certain other types of invaders.

Further inward—though still considered an *external* protective barrier—are the linings of the gastrointestinal tract (leading into the stomach) and the respiratory tract (leading to the lungs). In these linings are tiny, hair-like projections called *cilia*—which, like miniature brooms, sweep away any debris—and mucus, which traps bacteria and is then excreted. The stomach lining also protects itself by excreting hydrochloric acid.

There are, however, just too many destructive microorganisms in our environment for a simple mechanical barrier to cope, at least not without help from some sort of cellular intervention. As the British physician and comedian Jonathon Miller once said, "There are more microbes *per person* than the entire population of the world. Imagine that. Per person!" Without the vigilance of the immune system, these microbes and other microorganisms could easily destroy us through infection and disease. Consider how quickly the body decays after death,[1] when there is no longer a workable immune system left to ward off invaders and protect the integrity of the self.

In this chapter, we will delve deeper into the ways our immune systems protect us from the many "invaders" in our environment.

## VIGILANCE AND SAFETY

The immune system, at its most basic level, is easy to observe. We've all, at one time or another, seen and felt an immune-system reaction—after cutting a finger on a tin can, for instance, when bacteria from its surface have entered the wound. The cut and the area surrounding it swell up and become pink, hot, and painful to the touch. If the infection gets bad, it's not uncommon to find body temperature rising.

This process is called the *acute-phase reaction*, and it is the most basic, primitive first step that your immune system takes in its defense of you. The tiny troops it sends into the area are called *macrophages*. Macrophages (literally meaning "big eaters") and their tiny counterparts, *microphages,* are nonspecific defenders that your body sends at the first sign of an invasion, such as any bacteria or other foreign particles that got in as a result of that cut finger or scrape. These "scavenger cells," as they're called, are there as a first line of defense (see the inset "The Discovery of the Scavenger Cells" on page 20). They destroy and munch up any outsiders they find—except it's not called eating when macrophages do it; it's called *phagocytosis*.

## NONSPECIFIC IMMUNITY

There are several kinds of scavenging eater cells, or *phagocytes*, coursing around in your body, but the primary ones are microphages and macrophages. *Microphages*, the smaller ones, are of two kinds: *leukocytes*, or white cells (*leuko* means "transparent" or "white" in Greek, and *cyte* is the Greek word for "cell") and *granulocytes* (so called because within the cell one can see granules or grains). Microphages originate in the bone marrow, enter the bloodstream, circulate for a few days, then die. They're known as a form of *nonspecific immunity* because they don't really discriminate: they're like security guards, prowling around looking for trouble. What kind of trouble attracts them? Well, sometimes it's the microbes and microorganisms that have penetrated inside the body through a nick or cut; that invasion brings out a type of granulocyte called a *neutrophil*, which zooms over from where it's been hanging around in the bloodstream and "neutralizes" the invader. Macrophages and neutrophils are also part of the cause of inflammation, or swelling and tenderness. These cells migrate toward veins and capillaries and attach themselves to the coverings of these blood vessels at the site of injury.[2]

## HOT AND BOTHERED

Inflammation is, in and of itself, a safety device. Set in motion by a physical trauma or damage to tissues, it serves to "wall off" the injured area from undamaged sites. We've all seen it happen, often within seconds, after we've stubbed a toe or banged ourselves on something: the site swells up, gets red, feels hot to the touch, and

# The Discovery of the Scavenger Cells

*The amoeba-like cells that engulf foreign bodies, such as bacteria, were discovered nearly 100 years ago by a Ukrainian zoologist and microbiologist, Elie Metchnikoff (1845–1916), whose main area of interest, appropriately enough, was eating and digestion. Metchnikoff began his career as a professor of zoology and comparative anatomy at the University of Odessa in Russia. A few years later, in 1882, Metchnikoff was in Italy, off the coast of Sicily, and decided to collect some larvae from a species of small, transparent starfish. He took them back to his laboratory, put them under a microscope, and introduced some splinters and particles of carmine dye into them. Then Metchnikoff watched in amazement as a bunch of cells that were totally unconnected to the digestive system proceeded to eat the dye and splinters. Not exactly sure what he was witnessing, he then pricked the primitive creature with a small thorn. He saw the starfish "defend" itself against the invading thorn with a group of pugnacious and warlike macrophages.[1]*

*Metchnikoff decided to call these tiny eaters phagocytes (from "phagocytosis," meaning ingestion, or eating), a name that persists to this day. These tiny, swooping vacuum-cleaner cells became the early basis for the modern study of immunology.*

*Metchnikoff's discovery did not go unrewarded; he went on to become the director of the Bacteriological Institute in Odessa and in 1908 received (along with another pioneer of immunology, Paul Erhlich) the Nobel Prize for Physiology or Medicine for this essential immune-system discovery. (Metchnikoff appears to have become a little eccentric in his old age. In 1888, he went off to the Pasteur Institute in Paris, where he worked until his death in 1916 on a "fountain of youth" drug, trying to make lactic acid-producing bacteria increase longevity.)*

hurts. This is a protective mechanism: if you smash your foot against something, the swelling makes you limp, which automatically keeps the weight off it.

The scientific descriptions of inflammation haven't changed much through the centuries. It was first described in ancient times by Celcus, a Roman physician in the first century AD, as possessing four basic symptoms: heat, redness, swelling, and pain. There isn't a lot to be added by more recent explanations, other than that inflammation causes some loss of function. But today we do know the reasons: heat is produced by increased blood flow; redness is due to dilated blood vessels, swelling is caused mainly by cellular debris, and pain occurs partly as a result of the inflammation itself (acting on nerve endings) and partly because of chemical substances that are part of the inflammation process.[3]

The process of inflammation involves, first, a brief narrowing of the tiny blood vessels near the injury site, followed very quickly by the dilation, or widening, of the same blood vessels. Blood then rushes through them, and neutrophils attach themselves to the sides and then penetrate the vessel walls. Meanwhile, pus—made up of fluid, leukocytes, and cellular debris—collects. Normally, blood vessels allow fluid to pass through them freely, but inflammation traps fluid, causing edema (fluid retention) and permitting the neutrophils to stay on site and destroy the trapped bacteria and the damaged cells.

In addition, more microphages arrive and "sniff out" damaged tissue—much as reconnaissance crews search for signs that an enemy's been there by checking for fire damage or a blown-up building.

But although these microphage foot soldiers are pretty tough, they tend to work in a hand-to-hand combat kind of way, and their efforts don't always meet with total success. Some invaders have their own weapons, toxins that poison immune cells and render them powerless. Other microbes are bigger or just not digestible. By themselves, then, microphages are vulnerable; they need backup. This comes from the larger, more "muscular" macrophages.

Like their smaller, faster counterparts, macrophages also come from bone marrow and circulate in the blood. But they're fewer in number and slower, so rather than racing around in the bloodstream, they settle in lymphoid tissue, mostly in the spleen (on the left side of your abdomen) and in the lymph nodes scattered all over your body. (See Figure 2.1 on page 23.) In general, those pathogens that enter your system via the skin drain into local lymph nodes, and these are the nodes that become swollen and "active" when there is an infection close by. For instance, when you have a sore throat, you'll notice that the lymph nodes in your neck, closest to the site of the infection, have become inflamed. *Antigens*—substances that your immune system reacts to—that get in through your bloodstream, on the other hand, are usually attacked in the spleen.

Maybe because they're larger and "lazier," macrophages live longer than the microphage granulocytes. But if there's trouble, these macrophages do bestir themselves, and they do get there—not as fast as the quick microphages, but efficiently enough. Once they're there, these large cells attack the invaders using their own special kind of ammunition, a protein called interleukin-1 (IL-1), a term you may have heard in the medical news in recent years. Interleukin-1 stimulates liver cells to secrete another set of proteins that, via the bloodstream, get to the infected site, attach themselves to the products released by dying tissue cells, and assist in their harmless disposal. This process elevates temperature and enhances the immune response, thus assisting in the repair of damage. You can see this with the naked eye: first the cut is hot and infected, then pus develops and washes away impurities, and finally the site heals until there's nothing visible but a tiny scar (and sometimes not even that). When an inflammation becomes chronic, it is because the macrophages have for some reason failed to rid the site of the irritant or microorganism that was causing the problem.[3]

## VIRUSES: MINUTE INVADERS

Viral invasions are responded to just as quickly as are tissue dam-

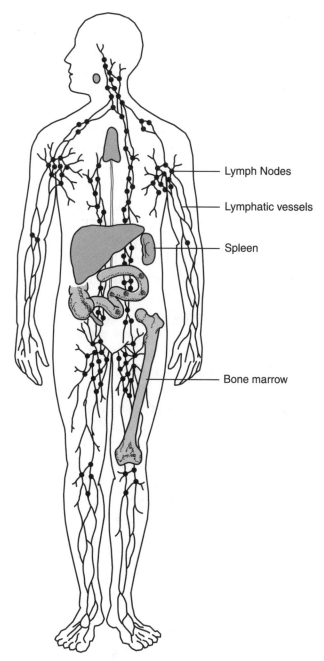

**Figure 2.1**. The lymphatic system.

age and trauma, but with different troops. Within hours after a virus has entered your body, macrophages produce interferon—another term you may have heard in the medical news in recent years. Interferon-1, the substance in question, works like an industrial spy who has infiltrated a rival organization. Essentially, what it does is throw a cellular monkey wrench into the workings of the virus, preventing it from reproducing. This buys time—the week or ten days it takes until more sophisticated cellular troops can get into the act.

The word *virus* comes from a Latin word meaning "slimy liquid" or "poison." Although historical descriptions of viral diseases date back to the tenth century, it was not until the late nineteenth century that more or less simultaneous experiments on tobacco plants by a Russian scientist, Dmitry Ivanovsky, and a Dutch scientist, Martinus W. Beijerinck, finally identified viruses.[4] Viruses were first noted for their tiny size: they could pass through a fine filter that would trap bacteria. It was then realized that these infectious microorganisms had to be different from bacteria, since they were not visible under a light microscope nor could they be cultured, as bacteria could, through artificial means.

Viruses are amazingly small. They range in size from 20 to 400 nanometers in size (by contrast, the smallest bacteria are about 400 nanometers)[5] and can multiply only in the living cells of animals, plants, or bacteria. (A nanometer is one-billionth of a meter.) Consisting mainly of protein, viruses are usually surrounded by single- or double-stranded nucleic acid (as in DNA); some also have an outer shell of fat. Outside of a living cell, a virus is inert, dormant; but once inside an appropriate host, it becomes a powerhouse of activity that takes over the host cell's metabolic machinery in order to create more viruses and reproduce itself.

Smallpox, herpes, influenza, and the common cold are caused by viruses, and in recent years it's been discovered that many other conditions can be *provoked* by viruses. A "simple" viral infection can lead to acute cardiac disease—requiring heart transplantation—or to Guillain-Barré syndrome, an acute autoimmune disorder, characterized by *febrile polyneuritis* (inflammation of many nerves), which almost invariably begins with a flu-like infection that then turns deadly.

Although viruses were originally described in terms of the diseases they caused, most viruses are not in and of themselves harmful. It is the *interaction* between the virus and its human host that creates a reaction, and it is the reaction that causes illness. Almost any virus can remain dormant in the tissues of the host: this is called *latency* and is the reason why some people who do not themselves develop symptoms of an illness may still be carriers of it.

Viral infections can have four different kinds of effects: (1) *inapparent*, whereby the virus lives in the host and produces no reaction; (2) *cytopathic*, in which the cell dies; (3) *hyperplastic*, in which the cell divides before dying, causing the immune system to react; and (4) *cell transformation*, wherein the cell not only divides but takes on an abnormal growth pattern and becomes cancerous.[6] A further, less understood response is one the immune system makes to certain viruses (and bacteria) known as *superantigens*, which have the ability to stimulate an immune response far beyond the normal. Unlike standard antigens, which bind to a single cell "marker," superantigens connect in two places. That may not seem like much, but what it does is to aggravate the immune system into mounting a full-scale, somewhat inappropriate response—a bit like sending thousands of untrained troops to fight a small group of terrorists when a smaller group of well-trained commandos would be more effective.[7] In theory, this should stop the enemy in its tracks; in reality, what often happens is that there is an unacceptably high degree of collateral, or secondary, damage to the body's own cells, which causes subsequent lingering physical problems. This self-inflicted damage can be severe, and there is some evidence that this collateral damage lies at the root of many autoimmune disorders. Multiple sclerosis, for example, is believed to result from one or more such viral infections.[8]

Some of the worst diseases in human history, including polio and smallpox, are caused by viruses. Since viruses live only within body cells, developing a drug that would kill only the virus and not damage the host's body tissues is virtually impossible. It was, therefore, the discovery of vaccines and immunization, and their widespread use, that was largely responsible for the eradication or near-eradication of these diseases. This will be covered in the next chapter.

From the discovery of the most primitive cellular defenses, the eater cells or phagocytes, to the widespread use of sophisticated vaccines took nearly a century. We have learned much more about the immune system in recent years. Before Dr. Ghoneum's MGN-3 could be discovered, however, a deeper understanding of the various cells that make up the immune system was necessary.

# Chapter 3

# Vaccination and Cellular Specifics

*"It is in moments of illness that we are compelled to recognize that we live not alone but chained to a creature of a different kingdom, whole worlds apart, who has no knowledge of us and by whom it is impossible to make ourselves understood: our body."*

—Marcel Proust (1871–1922), French writer

The reason we were all lined up as children and marched into the nurse's office for our vaccinations is that, in addition to the nonspecific responses that we generate at the threat of a foreign "invasion," our immune system has another card up its sleeve: specific, or acquired, immunity. True, the scavenging microphages and macrophages work amazingly well—and quickly, most of the time—but they react to all invaders in more or less the same way. If the danger persists, the immune system has to zap a target more intelligently, with a more specific, targeted response. The immune system has this ability in the form of an adaptive cellular immunity—also known as specific or acquired immunity—which doesn't quit after its initial, general response, but zeroes in on viruses, bacteria, or other harmful intruders with deadly accuracy.

When you think about it, this makes sense: your body can't possibly prepare itself for every kind of assault it's likely to encounter in a lifetime. So, by necessity, its first line of defense has to be a sort of scatter-gun approach. Often this nonspecific immune approach is enough. But when it's not, after a certain length of time, the immune system sends in bigger, or at least more accurate, guns. That's what specific, or acquired, immunity provides. More than just a tough thug, this immunological function is also smart. It remembers a former attack and keeps blueprints of what it was like in case it happens again. In this way, the body remembers how to react to something it has encountered before, even if the experience isn't exactly the same but only marginally similar. (See the inset "The Story of the Smallpox Vaccine" on page 29, which illustrates this point.)

In order to understand this aspect of our immune system, we need to know about some specific kinds of cells known as lymphocytes, which include T cells, cytotoxic T lymphocytes, and B cells. Once their cellular-specific functions are clear, we'll cover another efficient immune-system component—the natural killer cell. Then we'll see what happens when the immune reaction itself starts causing problems.

## LYMPHOCYTES—SMART BOMBS

As we saw in the previous chapter, the front-line response of the immune system is innate, rapid, and nonspecific. Like an emergency room at a large city hospital, it quickly deals with problems and stems the flow—much as the doctors and nurses in the ER do what they can to keep people alive until they can be transferred to the appropriate treatment area. But lurking behind that general area lie specific immune functions. Slower, not as quick to pick a fight, this cellular branch of the immune system consists of *lymphocytes* (so named because they primarily rest and are coded in the lymph nodes). These cells have the ability to recognize antigens (foreign particles that stimulate the immune system into forming an antibody), through a form of 3-D "vision." The great pioneer of immunology, Paul Ehrlich, described the actions of these cells as being like a key fitting into a lock; it's a fairly accurate picture, if one imagines both the key and the lock as being

# The Story of the Smallpox Vaccine

*Perhaps the most famous virus in the history of the immune system is variola, or smallpox. Disfiguring, highly infectious, and often fatal, smallpox would begin with symptoms similar to those of the flu and continue with a rash that spread all over the body. The rash would then turn into pus-filled blisters that became crusted and left its victims with ugly scars—if they survived. Complications from smallpox included blindness, pneumonia, and kidney damage.*

*Always widespread (once started, the contagious virus would spread like wildfire), smallpox reached epidemic proportions in eighteenth-century Europe. Over a forty-year period, it killed or disfigured close to 25 percent of the population in England alone. By the end of the 1700s, the public was clamoring for something to be done. They needed a safe method of inoculation.*

## VARIOLATION—A PRIMITIVE FORM
## OF INOCULATION

*Smallpox was widespread throughout most of human history. In certain parts of the East, like China, India, and Turkey, a primitive form of inoculation called variolation (where we get the name for the smallpox virus, variola) was practiced. The procedure involved scraping some pustules off a person infected with smallpox and then inoculating a healthy person with it through a tube inserted in the nose. This procedure, as disgusting as it sounds, did work but also carried some risks. (Later, it was done through the skin.) The practice of variolation was based on fairly solid evidence. It was known that a person who had once had the disease rarely would succumb to it a second time—due to a phenomenon known as acquired immunity—so it stood to reason that a person deliberately infected with a mild case of the disease would then be protected.*

Lady Mary Wortley Montagu (1689–1762) was one of the most brilliant, eccentric, and versatile women of her times. Born to a noble family, she refused the marriage her father had arranged for her and eloped with Wortley Montagu, a Whig, or liberal, member of Parliament. Montagu's party eventually came to power, and in 1716 he was appointed the British ambassador to Turkey. It was when the couple was in Istanbul that Lady Mary first became aware that Eastern medicine had a number of options Western medicine did not. In particular, she noticed that the Turks used something called variolation in an attempt to control smallpox. Smallpox interested Lady Mary a great deal; she herself had been severely stricken with smallpox in her youth and still bore the scars. Back in England a few years later in 1721, Lady Mary pioneered the practice of variolation against smallpox. (She later left her husband for an Italian count, but that's another story.)

Inoculating against smallpox using variolation techniques was, of course, better than nothing, but as a solution it lacked finesse. The person who was receiving it had, of necessity, to be healthy, but the disease's unpredictability could make it danger-ous. The transmitted disease did not always remain mild, and the inoculated person ran the risk not only of catching the virus but of passing it on to others. In addition, many physicians and reli-gious groups were firmly opposed to it.

### BIRTH OF THE MODERN SMALLPOX VACCINE

Enter Edward Jenner (1749–1823), a young British physician. Born at a time when medicine was gradually undergoing a shift and clinical work was becoming more "respectable," Jenner, after apprenticing for eight years with a practicing surgeon, moved to London. There, under the tutelage of some of the finest surgeons of the day, he developed his interests in anatomy, physiology, and experimentation.

*The son of a clergyman, Jenner always loved nature and during most of his career worked in small towns. Even as an apprentice, Jenner had noticed something peculiar: people who had been exposed to cowpox, a mildly eruptive disease that cows get on their teats, didn't seem to contract smallpox. Dairymaids, for instance, who milked the cows, would often get a mild form of cowpox and develop a rash on their hands, but they did not succumb to smallpox (which is where we get the notion of dairymaids having lovely skin; they didn't have the disfigurement and scarring of smallpox). Could this point to a safer means of inoculating people against smallpox?*

*In 1796, Jenner found a young dairymaid, Sarah Nelmes, who had fresh cowpox lesions on her finger. He took scrapings from the lesions and, on May 14, he used them to inoculate an eight-year-old boy. The boy promptly developed a slight fever and a low-grade lesion. Then, on July 1, he inoculated the boy again, this time with smallpox. But the boy didn't develop the disease.[1] And so the vaccine—the word is from the Latin word for "cow," vacca—was born.*

*The idea didn't take the world by storm. Jenner published his findings in 1797 in a slim volume called "An Inquiry into the Causes and Effects of the Variolae Vaccine, a Disease Known by the Name of Cow Pox," which was mostly ignored. But, eventually, the procedure proved its value and spread throughout the world.*

*As recently as thirty years ago, up to 15 million people annually were infected with smallpox (of whom 2 million died); but after ten years and some $313 million spent on vaccination, smallpox was declared eradicated for good.[2] In 1996, exactly 200 years after Jenner discovered the smallpox vaccine and twenty years after the last case (in Somalia), the World Health Organization declared that the last vial of this once-dreaded disease would soon be destroyed.*

made of modeling clay or another flexible substance.[1] But these observations don't give us a real sense of the immune system's full biological complexity.

A more complete description of how the antibody-antigen interaction works came in the late 1950s from the work of a Danish scientist, Niels Jerne (1911–1994), who was awarded the Nobel prize in 1984 for his work in immunology. Jerne envisioned an immune system of staggering diversity, one where individual cells were each programmed to recognize only a handful of antigens. Like a huge orchestra, all of whose members play music but each of whom plays a different instrument, these cells would respond only to those antigens that they alone could counter. This "network theory" that Jerne envisioned says that immune-system cells, through a form of cloning, alter themselves to meet whatever invader comes on the scene—and shut themselves off when they're not needed.[2]

After initial contact with an antigen, this adaptive branch of the immune system keeps a record of the attack and makes an antibody to go with it. In doing so, it acquires the necessary data to completely quash another attack from the same source should there ever be one. (Remarkably, a full description of how this acquired system works has only been around for the past few decades, even though we've known of its existence and how to stimulate it through vaccinations for a long time.)

Antigens are typically small "chunks" of intruding viruses or bacteria that bind to specific immune-system receptor cells. If they provoke a response, then we call them *immunogens*. In contrast, those antigens that can go up to a lymphocyte, shake its hand, and *not* provoke an immune response are called *haptens*—from the Greek word meaning "to grasp." Of course any relationship can turn sour, and a hapten can become immunogenic under certain circumstances (which is why immunologists often use haptens to study various immune reactions). What the immune system responds to is a particular pattern that the invading antigen has that is recognizable to specific lymphocytes.

Lymphocytes are in general a sleepy population, and unless they are signaled in some way, they don't react. But their numbers are enormous. At any given time, an adult person has billions of these lymphocytes, only about 1 percent of which are actually in the bloodstream.[3] Most of them lie in tissues like that of the bone marrow, spleen, thymus, lymph nodes, tonsils, and the lining of the intestines. There, they are confined to fine networks of tissue that channel them into contact with other cells, particularly our old friend the big eater, or macrophage. This ensures that lymphocytes do their battles in true military fashion: with order and precision.

Lymphocytes make up somewhere between 28 percent and 42 percent of all white blood cells. Most of them are small, with a huge nucleus that takes up most of their interior space. The two main types are B and T lymphocytes (often referred to as B cells and T cells). These two kinds of lymphocytes are indistinguishable and impossible to tell apart even under a microscope; it is only through their different functions that we are able to differentiate between them.

## T Cells—The Sharpshooters

T lymphocytes, or T cells, are called that because they go to a kind of military school in the thymus gland, located just behind the breastbone. There they start out as raw cadets, then mature, multiply, and develop different functions until they're ready to be called into action.

Helping the main army of killer T cells are two specialized subgroups called helper T cells (also identified as CD4) and suppressor T cells (also identified as CD8), which, as their names suggest, either enhance or reduce the killing power of the T cells. With the assistance of these helper cells, the killer T cells have remarkable accuracy: they can zero in, like sharpshooters, on an infected cell that's right next to a normal cell and destroy it—but leave the uninfected one alone.

## Cytotoxic T Lymphocytes

Cytotoxic T lymphocytes (CTLs) are so called because they share many of the characteristics of the T cell. CTLs recognize and respond to specific foreign antigens found on the surface of cancer cells, virus-infected cells, and other target cells. The CTLs then attach themselves to these antigens and destroy the target cells through a process called *CTL-induced lysis*, which involves injecting the unwelcome cells with destructive chemicals. In *in vitro* studies, this highly specific, powerful, rapid process occurs in about five hours.

## The B-Cell Army

B cells create a separate substance called *antibodies* (also referred to as *immunoglobulins*) that circulate through the fluids—what used to be called *humors*—in your body, providing you with what's called *humoral immunity*. On meeting a foreign invader, the B cells transform themselves into plasma cells, which, in turn, secrete immunoglobulins (Ig). Many pathogens, disease-causing toxins and microorganisms, are quickly neutralized and rendered harmless by the simple attachment of antibodies. For instance, the bacteria that cause tetanus (what you get from stepping on a rusty nail) become harmless when antibodies such as immunoglobulin G (IgG) stick to them.

There are five classes of immunoglobulins. IgG, IgM, and IgA are involved in humoral immunity (the actual destruction of the pathogen is usually left for the macrophages and granulocytes, which can do the job more efficiently). IgD is an immunoglobulin whose exact function remains unknown. IgE is the immunoglobulin active in allergies or hypersensitivities.[4] About 70 to 80 percent of the antibodies in our bloodstream are IgG; between 5 and 10 percent are IgM.[5]

T cells, in contrast, directly attack the foreign body. They are responsible for the body's rejection of transplanted tissue, for instance (see the inset "When the Immune System Misses the Point" on page 35).

## T Cells and B Cells Working Together

T cells help B cells along in their immunoglobulin-forming actions through a hormone-like substance called interleukin (IL). To date, sixteen varieties of interleukin have been discovered, with different and sometimes overlapping effects, and the end is not yet in sight. Interleukin-1 is secreted by macrophages, as you will remember, but helper T cells assist the B cells by calling on slightly different kinds of interleukin messengers—IL-2, IL-3, IL-4, and so on.[6] This cooperative effort is referred to as *cell-mediated immunity*. B and T cells work well together, though they perceive different things as threats that need to be attacked. In general, B cells are

---

# When the Immune System Misses the Point

*Many modern-day medical "miracles," like heart transplants and even some cosmetic surgeries, sometimes have disastrous consequences. The surgical process of taking one person's heart, lung, or kidney and transplanting it into someone else is actually a very straightforward procedure—at least, the mechanics of the surgical process are straightforward. But the individual dynamics are infinitely complex. Within moments, the recipient's immune system mounts a massive attack on the grafted or transplanted tissue, realizing that it's alien, not-self. Extremely powerful methods are required to suppress these graft-versus-host, or GVH, reactions; immunosuppressants such as cyclosporin and prednisone are routinely given to transplant patients. What this means is that these individuals, almost—though not quite—like people with AIDS, must take great care not to expose themselves to unnecessary risks. These immunologically fragile people may even find that going into a crowded mall presents an unacceptably high health risk.*

antibacterial, whereas T cells deal with more virulent threats, like cancer. But there they have help.

## NATURAL KILLER CELLS

Somewhere between the two types of protection (specific and non-specific) lies a particularly efficient type of cells called natural killer, or NK, cells. Like the ruthless terrorists that we so often see in thrillers, NK cells are programmed to kill tumor cells on sight and ask questions later. They don't care about the whys and wherefores; they're small, they're armed (with granules inside the cell that, like bullets, charge into the cancer cell and destroy it), and they're dangerous. (See Figure 3.1.) NK cells were first discovered in 1975 when researchers observed cells in the blood that appeared to be neither scavenger cells nor lymphocytes, but were nevertheless able to kill tumor cells *in vitro* (literally, "in glass"; usually in a test tube or flask). They look like lymphocytes, except for those granules inside. (In fact, they are now considered to be a type of lymphocyte.) And they have an unerring instinct to kill (most of the time) and to zero in on cancer, or tumor, cells in particular. Somehow, they bind to these cells and "shoot" them dead.

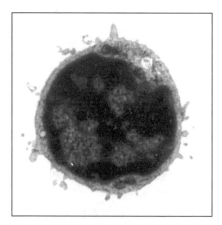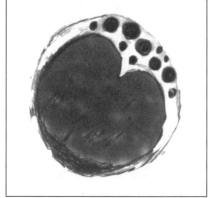

**Figure 3.1.** A single natural killer (NK) cell. A light micrograph of an NK cell is on the left, and an illustration of an NK cell is on the right.

Another kind of killer cell—called a K cell or a lymphokine-activated killer (LAK) cell—may be either a variant of the NK cell or some kind of lymphocyte, which it physically resembles. These killers have receptors that bind to the free end of a chain of immunoglobulin G; the side that's not attached to the antigen. (IgG and IgA, along with lymphocytes, are the most common responses to a threat.) It's like catching on to the end of the string that is *not* attached to the bomb. Once there, at the end of the "string," the NK cells appear to function like SWAT team explosives experts: K cells inject into the IgG chain a lethal substance, the exact nature of which remains unknown, that causes the cell to swell and explode.

Given the shoot-first-ask-questions-later tendencies of these killer cells, the immune system needs to control them in some way; otherwise they would destroy everything around them. And it does through the use of *cytokines,* chemical messengers that prevent the immune response from overreacting—although in certain autoimmune disorders it appears that the cytokines are actually the cause of the immune system's attacking the person's own tissue.

## RECOGNIZING THE ENEMY

How does the immune system tell the difference between an enemy and a harmless invader? That varies between people, but, basically, *immunocompetence*—the biological sense of what is self and what is not—originates very early, before birth and in the months just after birth. Breastfeeding a baby enhances immunocompetence immensely, since at birth we are relatively helpless against many common pathogens, and there are antibodies in breast milk. A 1990 Scottish study that tracked 668 babies found, for instance, that breastfed babies had far fewer stomach problems than bottle-fed ones.[7]

At this early point, any cells that are *autoreactive* (programmed to react and kill cells that are self) are eliminated. Early lymphocytes are "called" to the thymus gland, located just below the thyroid at the front of the neck. But though many are called, few are chosen for action. The cells that are destined to recognize self are kept on, and the rest are destined to sit on the sidelines, never called into action.

On the flip side of the equation, a foreign particle presented early enough to the immune system can become incorporated into "self" and will not be perceived as foreign. That was neatly demonstrated in a 1953 experiment by a famous immunologist, Peter Medawar, who discovered that if a newborn white mouse was injected with cells from a black mouse, the white mouse's immune system was tricked into believing it was "black" as well.[8] Skin grafts from the black mouse could be transplanted onto the white mouse without fear of rejection. Medawar's experiment is a further indication of the complexity of the immune system: only the cells destined to be useful in the protection and reproduction of the self survive, and the rest are rendered inactive, inert, or nonreactive.

The cellular individuation process is called *histocompatibility*. It works as a marker—something like a bar code—that tells your lymphocytes what belongs and what does not. As techniques to match histocompatibility have become more sophisticated, and researchers have learned to "type" tissues through matching histocompatibility antigens for the donor and the recipient, the success of organ transplantation has been vastly improved.

The "bar code" information consists of a coating of molecules on normal cells that tells your immune system what is okay and what is not. These identifying molecules are known as *major histocompatibility complex* (MHC) antigens, and you will read more about them in later chapters; they are critically important for AIDS patients, among others.

## REMEMBERING THE ATTACK

Amazingly, once an immune-system attack has taken place and antibodies have formed in reaction to some invading microorganism, not all the antibodies to that pathogen disappear. Some linger. In a way, it's like leaving some troops for peacetime endeavors after a war has been won. This is the immune system's "memory." Once it has been exposed to something, it files away the information. This way, if that particular antigen shows up again, it'll know

tion. This way, if that particular antigen shows up again, it'll know what to do. Therein lies the idea of an adaptive, acquired specific immunity. With organ transplants, if a person rejects a kidney or a heart with one kind of antigenic marker, a second organ with the same type of marker will be rejected faster and more violently. Similarly, bad allergic reactions don't happen the first time someone is exposed to a substance, but the second—and each subsequent time, the reaction is stronger. It is also the reason vaccination is effective: once exposed to a mild version of a disease, a person is less likely to get sick from it again. The immune system mounts a powerful response and repels the attack.

Unfortunately, these processes don't always work as well as we used to think they did. Vaccinations do not confer lifetime immunity as was once believed, but only for fifteen to twenty years. What researchers who studied the immune system at the turn of the century assumed would remain a fail-safe defensive system actually gets its wires crossed, misses important signals, and even targets the wrong cells at times—much as a large army, through miscommunication, bureaucratic bungles, or other errors (usually called "human error" in the subsequent inquiries!) can miss the intended target.

## WHEN THE IMMUNE SYSTEM BECOMES THE ENEMY

At other times, problems can arise when the immune system is just doing its job. The normal response to a foreign body can become harmful, leading to tissue damage or, on occasion, creating dangerously high levels of the by-product of this process, called *cytokines*. Cytokines are biologically active proteins that are not intruder- or antigen-specific.[9] Usually, they are important regulators of the immune system and help communicate information back and forth. But, for unknown reasons, there are times when they reproduce too quickly. Much in the same way as the weapons used in the Gulf War led to Gulf War syndrome, leaving many troops with lingering health after-effects, an immune-system attack can have negative consequences.

Metchnikoff's macrophages were indeed walling off and attempting to destroy the invading thorn (see the inset "The Discovery of the Scavenger Cells" on page 20), but there are several situations—tuberculosis (TB) is one—where it is the immune reaction itself that causes the problem. In TB, it is the macrophage that serves as the host or the "home" for the bacterium. It creates a "capsule" for it. This, in turn, is attacked by the immune system— which gives the immune system the capacity to injure as well as heal.[10] Many, if not most, viral diseases (acute, short-term ones like the flu and chronic, long-term ones like herpes) are often not a direct effect of the virus itself but of the secondary immune response.[11] The virus, once recognized as immunologically foreign, is attacked in one of two ways: through an antibody attack or via a direct frontal attack from an immune cell. It is the former, the antibody attack, that can destroy parts of the person as well as the virus. Different individuals are genetically predisposed toward one of these types of immune reaction, so those people who are physiologically inclined not to make antibodies are very susceptible to bacterial infections but usually don't get colds or other viral infections.[12]

Scientists have not yet reached an understanding of the extent to which pollutants, chemical carcinogens, and the stress of modern life may have caused the immune system to get its wires crossed. We also don't know to what extent the immune system can become a victim of fatigue and overload, in the same way that a person who is overextended, overtired, and stressed can become more prone to accident, injury, and disease. But we do know that the immune system can be incapacitated or severely impaired by infections, malnutrition, stress, or exposure to toxic substances. At other times, the immune system can simply be overwhelmed by the severity of an attack. Before the discovery of antibiotics, many people died of diseases that are now no longer considered dangerous—and people continue to die of infections when their immune systems are overwhelmed.

In Chapter 4, we will examine the cause of most infections, bacteria, and trace a discovery that changed the face of Western medicine—antibiotics. We will also explore the reasons that antibiotic therapy is becoming less effective and the new directions in which medical practice is—slowly—beginning to move.

# Chapter 4

# Interacting With a Hostile World

*"Disease is very old, and nothing about it has changed. It is we who change, as we learn to recognize what was formerly imperceptible."*

— Jean Charcot (1825–1893), French neurologist

In biological terms, the human environment is actually a rather hostile one. The air we breathe, the soil we walk on, the waters and vegetation, and even the buildings we live in are all populated with microscopically small forms of life that are only too willing to invade us—since many of them must live off other living cells to survive.

We usually defend ourselves quite well against these threats; our immune system works around the clock to recognize what it needs to react to and what it can ignore. But when the immune system isn't up to the challenge, we need outside help—particularly if the attacking microorganism is an especially virulent one. In this chapter, we trace how human understanding of these microbes developed and where we are today in terms of dealing with these microscopic threats.

## A WORLD-CHANGING DISCOVERY

Bacteria, the most common form of microorganisms, are present on just about every surface—which explains all those television ads urging us to buy soap powders and bathroom sprays that have been especially formulated to kill bacteria. Many bacteria live and multiply on nonliving matter and are, therefore, easily transferable to humans. The history of surgery was mostly a history of death and dying until it was realized that the infections from which surgical patients died were caused by the invasion of bacteria from dirty surfaces into the wound.

The history of bacteriology mirrors closely the history of *microscopy*—development of the microscope—since it was the microscope that led to the discovery of bacteria. The first person to actually see bacteria was probably the Dutch naturalist Antonie van Leeuwenhoek, in 1683. (Leeuwenhoek was either not the most accurate of observers or blessed with a fantastic imagination: when he looked at sperm under the microscope, he "saw" tiny, anatomically perfect men inside them. However, he did correctly deduce that sperm were involved in reproduction.) Bacteria were visible under a lens that magnified about 100 to 150 diameters. But it was not until the late nineteenth century that their significance became known. An understanding of their connection to disease came about through a man we associate with milk: the French scientist Louis Pasteur, from whom we get the term *pasteurization*—the process of heating certain foods for a period of time to kill harmful bacteria, like those in raw milk.

Bacteria can be killed on surfaces with antiseptics and other disinfectants; unfortunately, these cannot be used on living tissue because in the necessary strengths they are far too toxic. An interesting form of virus, known as a bacterial virus or *bacteriophage*, also kills bacteria. It does this by attaching its own genetic material (DNA or RNA) to the bacterium and either taking over the cell's machinery or simply rendering it inactive. Bacteriophages—now also called *phages*—were discovered independently by two scientists: Frederick Twort in Great Britain in 1915 and Félix d'Hérelle in France in 1917. Phage therapy in humans was not found to be promising, and the discovery of antibiotics some years later led to the abandonment of research in this area. There has been a renewal of interest in this field in recent years, however, with the development of stronger, antibiotic-resistant bacteria. It's entirely possible that in the near future, antibiotic therapy will be replaced by a combination of gene therapy and bacteriophage therapy.

Another means of killing microorganisms is *sterilization*, by either high heat and pressure or a chemical agent, which kills all the bacteria on a particular surface. For many years, sterilization has been used to kill bacteria on surgical instruments. *Preservatives* are used mostly for keeping foods free of harmful organisms for a time; one of the oldest known preservatives is salt. Freezing also keeps organisms at bay.

Louis Pasteur's methods of vaccine production (see the inset "Louis Pasteur: An Avid Observer" on page 46) led to the rapid development of vaccines for many diseases, from whooping cough to diphtheria. By the mid-1950s, a number of these deadly diseases were controlled through vaccination. But Pasteur's vaccines, made by diminishing the strength of a bacterium *in vitro* and then using that as a vaccine, were not the only form of vaccine. Several different versions of the polio vaccine were introduced in this century before the Salk vaccine—which uses three separate viruses in a formalin-inactivated vaccine—was accepted. A typhoid vaccine developed by British bacteriologist Sir Almroth Wright (1861–1947) used *autogenous*—derived from the self—vaccines, prepared from bacteria harbored by the patient and rendered harmless through the application of heat. Wright tested his vaccine on thousands of soldiers in India. He was so successful at vaccinating British troops during the Boer War that Britain was the only combatant engaged in that war that did not lose more soldiers from infection than from firepower.[1]

Wright resigned from the army in 1902 and became a professor of pathology at St. Mary's Hospital in London. At that point, vaccines had gone a long way toward controlling and preventing disease, but it was the repercussions from Pasteur's work with bacte-

# Louis Pasteur: An Avid Observer

*Bacteria have been around a lot longer than humans, but it was-n't until the late nineteenth century that they managed to make the front pages of scientific news. Even though medicine had rec-ognized their role in disease, prior to the work of one man it was not known how such microscopic creatures could actually affect humans. Louis Pasteur (1822–1895) was an outstanding French chemist and microbiologist who single-handedly brought bacteria to the forefront of medicine, where they belonged.*

*Pasteur, who began his career as a high-school physics teacher, was an avid experimenter and observer. His first scientific paper, published when he was only twenty-six and had just received his Ph.D., was on tartaric acid—an acid formed when grapes ferment during the making of wine—and showed how certain compounds were capable of creating chemical mirror-images of each other. In 1863, Pasteur became the dean of the new science faculty at the University of Lille, in northern France, where he instigated the then-revolutionary idea of holding evening university classes that could be attended by working people. In Lille, Pasteur was approached by an industrialist with a question about the fermen-tation of grain and beet sugar. Again he encountered the mirror-image effect in certain chemicals, and from there he went on to observe that certain organisms—like yeast—could reproduce themselves, later known as the Pasteur effect.*

*Over time, Pasteur began to wonder whether, as was then believed, organisms "spontaneously" regenerated themselves, or if, instead, some microorganisms—bacteria—were simply always present in the environment. Using simple and precise experi-ments, Pasteur proved that bacteria were, indeed, present on all surfaces.*

*Today, we take it for granted that there are "germs" present on surfaces and in the air, but a century ago that knowledge revolu-tionized—and saved—many industries, including both the wine* industry and the silkworm industry, two mainstays of France's economy. Later, while conducting research for French and British breweries, Pasteur developed a process that prevented the rapid deterioration of beer—no doubt one of his more popular discoveries.

Although Pasteur was partially paralyzed in 1868 and officially retired, he kept busy. It was in his later years that he discovered a way to reduce the virulence of bacteria in order to produce a vaccine for anthrax, a disease that can ravage sheep and other domesticated animals. His most spectacular discovery was a vaccine for rabies. Pasteur found that by "culturing" bacteria, he could weaken them. He experimented with animals, then on his own children, and on July 6, 1885, he saved the life a nine-year-old boy who had been bitten by a rabid dog. The vaccine was an outstanding success.

ria—and their disease-causing properties—that was to truly change the face of medicine.

## HOW ANTIBIOTICS CHANGED THE FACE OF MEDICINE

In human beings, *infectious disease* is a process set in motion by the presence of minute microorganisms, usually bacteria. An *infection,* on the other hand, is the result of a direct invasion of the body by bacteria *and* the immune system's reaction to their presence. An infection that does not cause disease is said to be *subclinical,* or below the level of clinical detection or medical intervention. Thus, a person may be infected but not have an infectious disease—like Typhoid Mary, one of the most famous disease carriers in American history, who was infected with the bacterium *Salmonella typhi,* or typhoid.

Typhoid Mary's real name was thought to be Mary Mallon, and she was said to have come to the United States in 1870 (from where is not clear). More than fifty cases of typhoid and three

deaths in the New York area in the early 1900s were traced directly to homes where she'd worked as a cook—and countless more
cases were blamed on her. After some clever sleuthing on the part
of public health officials, she was discovered, only to disappear,
then reappear, again working as a cook. Finally, New York authorities, led by public sanitation officer George Soper, tracked her
down and had her committed to an isolation unit. There she stayed
until 1910, when the health department finally released her on condition that she not work with food again. She apparently ignored
that: four years later, after a typhoid outbreak in New Jersey, she
was found in the place where the typhoid had appeared. She was
apprehended again and kept in isolation until her death in 1932.

Unfortunately, at that time, the medical community did not
realize that a simple mold, *Penicillin notatum*, could kill the typhoid
bacillus, although herbalists and other "folk" medical practitioners
had known for a long time that certain molds could control infection. Gypsy women in Europe used moldy cabbage leaves to dress
wounds, for example. But it wasn't until 1928, when Alexander
Fleming was working as an aide in Sir Almroth Wright's laboratory in London, that laboratory proof of this mold's efficacy in killing
bacteria was made scientifically—and inadvertently.

Fleming discovered one day that colonies of bacteria growing
on a petri dish had been "killed" by a penicillin mold. The substance proved too unstable to be used clinically at that point, and
ten years passed before the primary ingredient in *Penicillin* was
identified. (Fleming shared the 1945 Nobel Prize for Medicine with
Ernst Chain and Howard Florey, both of whom also worked on
pinpointing the active substance in penicillin.) The drug was called
an *antibiotic*, after "antibiosis," a term used in the 1880s to describe
the destruction of one living being by another. It was first applied
to the treatment of infections in 1941. This simple discovery visibly
and abruptly changed the whole face of Western medicine, and
forever altered our view of disease.

Suddenly, disease was defined through an external cause—
microbes, a cause for which doctors could prescribe a drug. (As
one anonymous wag put it, in the nineteenth century men lost

their fear of God and acquired a fear of microbes instead.) Over time, as antibiotics became more sophisticated, more infections were added to the list of diseases that antibiotics could cure. Toward the end of the 1950s, scientists attached various chemical groupings to the penicillin core to generate semi-synthetic versions, and today there are high-tech antibiotics that can zero in on specific bacteria with fewer side effects than the early versions.

Penicillins kill the bacteria that cause strep throat, pneumonia, spinal meningitis, diphtheria, and syphilis through a "hacking" process, breaking down the cell walls of the bacteria and "neutralizing" the enzymes within the bacteria that are responsible for building the cell walls. They are therefore ineffective against any bacterium *without* a cell wall, such as the one responsible for tuberculosis. There, another form of antibiotic—streptomycin, identified in 1943—is used. It functions by disturbing the process that bacteria use to regenerate and multiply. Still other antibiotics (for instance, nystatin) affect the cell membranes of yeasts and fungi. But no antibiotic can kill a virus. (Alexander Fleming apparently was asked, at a news conference in 1954, what he did for a cold, and he suggested a shot of whisky at bedtime. "It's not very scientific," said the discoverer of penicillin, "but it helps.")

## TOO MUCH OF A GOOD THING?

In the relatively short time since antibiotics were discovered, both doctors and patients have become accustomed to thinking of them as a panacea, a solution to all forms of disease. Because antibiotics destroy the causes of some diseases, we have assumed that they work against *all* of them—which they do not. Furthermore, a major problem that has plagued antibiotic therapy since its very beginnings has been the resistance that bacteria can develop, quite quickly, to the drugs. An antibiotic may kill *most* of the disease-causing bacteria in the system of a person taking it, but there are always exceptions: a few tough bacteria that remain genetically less vulnerable. Those stronger bacteria then go on to reproduce and transfer their resistance to others—hence the frightening headlines we've all seen about "unkillable" antibiotic-resistant bacteria. Unfortunately, it is primarily through the indiscriminate and inexact use of antibiotics that resistance developed in the first place.[2] One of the highlights of the medical news in 1997 was that the bacterium *Staphylococcus aureus* showed resistance to vancomycin,[3] the lone remaining antibiotic that had been effective against it. This development, of course, should not come as a huge shock: as a culture, we have long been prone to overconsumption and excess, and it's no surprise that we ended up believing that there's no such thing as too much of a good thing.

The crux of the matter—at the time they were discovered and, to some extent, up to the present—is that antibiotics were the first therapy that medical science had to offer that actually worked. Prior to that and throughout most of human history, disease was largely mysterious, incomprehensible. How or why people got sick was unknown, and the origins of disease were shrouded in mysticism and magic. Illness was generally perceived as a foreign element lodged in the person's body, sometimes even associated with moral weakness. Vague terms like "distemper" and "the falling sickness" (presumably epilepsy) were used to describe illness. One man was said to be "consumed by a giant worm," and Charles II of Spain, dying in 1700, was believed to be bewitched. Therapy consisted mostly of easing symptoms with the few remedies available, like mercury, digitalis, ipecac root, and opium—the latter was addictive but at least useful in reducing pain. Physicians were trained in the classics but knew little of biology or organic life; they "prescribed, dosed, and bled, leaning on pedantic scholarship blended with primitive psychology."[4] They often did much less for people in terms of cure than could the local wisewoman or healer. As the Scottish physician William Cullen wrote: "We know nothing of the nature of contagion that can lead us to any measures for removing or correcting it. We only know its effects." That held true throughout most of human history. But suddenly, in the middle of the twentieth century, doctors had antibiotics—drugs that could actually *do* something, that could alleviate the symptoms of, and even cure, a bacterial infection.

## THE "MAGIC" OF MEDICINE

Despite our present sophistication with respect to how illness occurs, the very complexity and enormous availability of medical options in the Western world means that most of us are just as ignorant today about disease—albeit in a different way—than people in earlier centuries. So it makes sense that we've transformed pharmacotherapy (drug therapy), surgery, and other modern interventions into a kind of magic of our own age. Trust "the doctors" to fix whatever ails us, be it cancer or a cold.

Yet as studies by medical ethicists, sociologists, and other observers have noted, we pay a hefty price socially, emotionally, personally, and financially for our medical advances and expertise. Nobody dies a "natural" death any more; you die of cardiac arrest—usually in the hospital. Discussions about dying with dignity and physician-assisted suicide center on our fears that medical science will keep our bodies alive long after our spirit has died. The technology has surpassed our ability to cope with it.

Recent research is even calling into question the preventive and clinical benefits of widespread vaccination. Although there's no question that the eradication of diseases like smallpox and polio has been of enormous benefit, the evidence is growing that suppressing *all* childhood diseases may actually be counterproductive. Early immune stimulation through a bout of measles, mumps, or chickenpox actually may play an important part in adult health and in the healthy development of immunity. Immunity that's properly balanced, with the capacity to be neither too active—which could fling the person into autoimmune disorders—nor too passive, unable to fend off cancer and other diseases.

In the prestigious medical journal *The Lancet,* British physician Dr. Andrew Wakefield and his co-workers reported that most of a small group of children diagnosed with enterocolitis—inflammation of the colon, causing pain, diarrhea, and, on occasion, fever and loss of some developmental skills, including language—had had the MMR vaccine against measles, mumps, and rubella just before their symptoms began.[5] All the children had intestinal abnormalities and chronic inflammation of the colon; some showed evidence of autism, and one showed a possible postviral or vaccinal encephalitis. The authors suggest that "environmental triggers" might have been responsible for these children's conditions, and the one that leaps to mind, naturally, is the vaccination they had received. Doctors have rushed to say that this study is not conclusive, and they are right. It's not. But it does inject a note of doubt into a form of medical practice that was, for years, considered unassailably perfect.

## VACCINATION GONE WRONG

A more obvious case of vaccination gone wrong is the case of diphtheria in Russia. With the advent of a widely used vaccine against diphtheria in the 1950s, that disease underwent a sharp decline. In the Soviet Union, as in many places, cases of diphtheria were practically unheard of. But after the Soviet Union broke up into smaller states and vaccination was no longer routinely done, diphtheria came back with a vengeance. According to World Health Organization figures, over 90 percent of all diphtheria cases in the world occurred in this region. Why? Because the vaccine had virtually eradicated the organism that causes the disease. And because the protection conferred by vaccines is short-lived, twenty years at most, as many as 60 percent of adults had lost their immunity and were susceptible to the disease when vaccinations stopped and their children began to get diphtheria.[6] If they'd had the disease naturally, they would have been protected.

What the Russian example shows is that starting and then stopping broad-based vaccination programs can set in motion some ominous effects. Breaking the cycle of natural childhood disease—which would normally be followed by long-lasting immunity in those who survived to adulthood—through a vaccination program that is then stopped actually leaves adults *more* vulnerable to disease than they otherwise would have been.[7]

We do not mean to imply that vaccinations should be abandoned. On the contrary, we know full well that our longevity today is partly a result of people not dying at a young age from smallpox, polio, and other formerly common killers. There is also evidence, of course, that it is not medical advances alone that have brought about our longer life span but social and economic improvements like universal education, clean water, better nutrition, well-preserved food, and the addition of vitamins to staple foods.

## EXPLORING NEW CONCEPTS

Research is under way into artificially produced DNA (polynucleotide) vaccines, a new concept of immunization that holds enormous promise. The body will be stimulated to use this artificial DNA, which will be directly injected, to create a blueprint to manufacture proteins that stimulate the immune response.[8] Another research direction with major potential is an AIDS vaccine, which—even if it could prevent *some* of the new cases of AIDS each year—would be a substantial health benefit for the world. At present, new AIDS cases are rising at an alarming rate, especially in the developing world. In Zimbabwe, for instance, because of AIDS, the average life expectancy for a male is expected to drop to 49 (from 56) by the end of this century.[9] A vaccine might at least stem the tide.

But, overall, vaccines and other immune system–supported means of attaining health have not received the same medical attention in recent years as have pharmaceutical and surgical approaches. While drug companies may well have had a hand in this, the tide of medical "fashion" has also gone in the direction of eradication versus prevention. Changing technology, a popular culture dominated by the media, and extraordinary advances in everyday life—from fax machines to automatic bank tellers—have created a society unlike any other in human history. The prevailing ethos is based on a "fix it" approach, one that assumes that bodies, like anything else, can simply be repaired. A new heart—an artificial one, if need be—can be put in to replace a defective one.

But the immune system knows only too well what is self and what is not. Ever vigilant, it rejects high-tech solutions. The sheer numbers of people suffering from cancer, AIDS, autoimmune disorders, allergies, and other modern ailments indicate that a change in how we approach these problems is called for: a view that appreciates the enormous complexity of individuals and the diseases to which they are susceptible.

Unlike the bacteriological model—which assumes that disease is caused by a microorganism that can be destroyed with the appropriate antibiotic—using the immune system itself to fight disease requires finesse and individuation. It's complicated—and, as the Roman orator and statesman Cicero complained, "Physicians, when the cause of a disease is discovered, consider that the cure is discovered." In fact, most of the time it is not.

The immune system is an extremely complex network. In some ways, it is as if each of us has a minuscule universe inside us. Complicated biological actions, interactions, and reactions go on continually, with a dynamic flow that we are only beginning to recognize. And given the increasingly dangerous environment that we live in, full of pollutants—many of them carcinogens (cancer-causing substances)—a well-functioning immune system is more essential than ever. The problem is that we are in a race against time, struggling to find solutions to medical problems that threaten to engulf us.

Nevertheless, as information becomes more readily available on the Internet and through the media, as more people realize that the solutions are complex and multi-layered, we move toward a more rational view of health (or eliminating ill health). Alternative strategies, formerly the domain of a few cranks, have moved into the mainstream as more and more patients take matters of health into their own hands. In this climate, it would not be unreasonable to assume that we are finally going to realize the importance of a healthy immune system—and to propel immune research back into the forefront of medical science, where it was 100 years ago.

There are treatments on the market today that claim to strengthen the immune system. Because of its complexity, however, drugs—whether they are herbs or pharmaceuticals—that simply "boost" the immune system may do more harm than good. It is essential that any product that modulates immune-system function have solid scientific evidence behind it, as well as clinical trials (trials on human beings). In the next chapter, we will look at one such product, now known as MGN-3, and how it came to be used very effectively.

# Chapter 5

# Modulating the Immune System

*"Those who are enamored of practice without science are like a pilot who goes into a ship without rudder or compass and never has any certainty where he is going. Practice should always be based on a sound theory of knowledge."*

—Leonardo da Vinci (1452–1519), Italian artist, engineer, and scientist

The central role that the immune system plays in keeping illness at bay has been known for a long time. Unfortunately, medical science has never known exactly how to use this information. For one thing, each person's immune system is individual and reacts differently, even to the same virus. We all know people who succumb to every cold or flu that goes around while someone else sitting at the next desk doesn't seem to catch anything. Yet that same person who "never gets sick" may end up with something serious—like heart disease or cancer.

In recent years, a lot of press has been given to the idea of somehow "enhancing" or shoring up individual immunity. Market forces being what they are, various compounds, herbs, and other substances that promise to strengthen or, to put it more scientifically, modulate the immune system do a booming business. The problem is that very few of these actually tell you what part of the immune system they're purported to affect or what they really do.

As we saw in the preceding chapters, the immune system is enormously complex and has an extraordinary number of cellular functions, from general, scatter-gun approaches to specific, well-targeted responses. And, depending on the nature of the assault or "attack," the strength of the virus or bacterium, or the genetic predisposition of the person, immune response varies. So how exactly do we know that what we're taking to modulate our immune system is actually helping to achieve the desired goal? The short answer is that we usually don't. In healthy people who are simply trying to ward off a cold or not get sick, this probably isn't that big a deal. But for those who have something seriously wrong, this uncertainty can be hazardous.

## THE IMMUNE SYSTEM AND CANCER THERAPY

The notion that the immune system should be engaged in cancer therapy is gradually gaining ground, especially since standard cancer therapy—what some call "slash, burn, and poison"—can sometimes be worse than the disease. Despite the toxic effects of standard therapies, however, many patients do beat cancer and, having learned a lot about it, many have become activists in their own right. They've read books and attended lectures, worked to understand what is going on, taken matters into their own hands. They've written and spoken about their own battles with cancer and passed on what they've learned.

The media have been invaluable as well; every day another article or television news story lets people know about alternative and complementary therapies that have been shown to work. Even though the cancer establishment has steadfastly refused to acknowledge that pollution, toxic chemicals, and industrial waste may play a part in the development of cancer, people have rallied together and—through boycotts, demonstrations, and smart use of the media—have forced some industries to change or modify their practices. Medical authorities might recognize only that diet "may have something to do with" the development of cancer, but through the media and through books and lectures, committed individuals have succeeded in persuading millions of people to add more fruits and vegetables to their diet and have created a booming market in organic produce. All this bodes well for "patient power" in general. There is a downside, however, to that kind of public advocacy for alternative views of medical therapy.

## THE PROBLEM WITH ALTERNATIVE VIEWS

Unfortunately, many untested, unproven therapies of questionable merit can, with a good public relations campaign, become more widely known and used than remedies that are more effective but less "hyped." As a general rule, anything that's said to cure everything from snake bites to skull fractures should be viewed with skepticism if not outright dismay. It's simply not possible for one substance to work on *everything*.

Furthermore, nothing works on *everybody*. There is much too much human variability and idiosyncrasy. So when a drug or a treatment is said to "work," the phrase reflects a statistical reality rather than a 100-percent prediction. It works on most people, most of the time, for whatever it is supposed to fix. Even aspirin is not something everyone can take. This, of course, is true of standard therapies just as much as it's true of "alternative" or complementary treatments.

"Many of the products that are on the market have not been tested scientifically," says immunologist Dr. Mamdooh Ghoneum, Ph.D., chief of research in the Department of Otolaryngology (the branch of medicine that deals with the ear, nose, and throat) at Drew University of Medicine and Science in Los Angeles and an assistant professor in the UCLA Department of Neurobiology. "Scientific means that you have to start in the quantitative stages. Start with animals. Then you go to what we call *in vitro* studies (literally 'under glass,' or done in a test tube—in the laboratory, in other words)." Like a staircase, the process involves a series of steps that need to be followed; each successful stage leads to another.

## SENSIBLE SCIENCE

The term *alternative* is a somewhat strange one, given that it reflects merely what is generally accepted and what is not. The medical establishment often insists that alternative therapies lack scientific proof; yet, many alternative therapies have solid research behind them. And we've all seen so-called fringe therapies become mainstream after a certain amount of time. Acupuncture, for instance, as recently as fifteen years ago was considered by many doctors to be a curiosity at best, complete quackery at worst. But only a short time ago, the American Medical Association and various other medical groups declared acupuncture an effective treatment for certain types of pain and nausea. Anti-angiogenesis to shrink tumors—which is what shark cartilage does—was pooh-poohed for years; yet, only a few months ago, it was on the cover of national newsmagazines and headlined in major newspapers across the country.

Nevertheless, it's vital that individuals who want to embark on complementary therapeutic routes make sure that what they're about to take is safe and at least makes *sense*. A good rule of thumb is that if the substance in question is a "secret" known to only one person or institution, which cannot release the substance for scientific testing . . . well, that's probably not the most sensible route to take. You need to understand the source and the mechanism of whatever it is you're going to take, and decide whether it is reasonable or not.

## "BOOSTING" IMMUNITY

When it comes to the immune system, indiscriminately "boosting" it may end up doing more harm than good. In later chapters dealing with allergies and autoimmune disorders, you will see how dangerous such a course of action could be. "Any blanket recommendation to 'tone up' the immune system may prove to be bad advice," writes immunologist Mark Lappé.[1] "The alternative, to have tightly honed, [specific] immune responses tailored to individual tumor antigens, is just now being explored." It's important that any immune modulator—known as *biological response modifiers*, or *BRMs*, in the scientific community—have behind it solid scientific evidence and clinical trials with proof that it works. It's only too easy to prey on sick, desperate people who feel abandoned by the medical community and who are clutching at straws.

## THE DISCOVERY OF MGN-3

Dr. Mamdooh Ghoneum, a soft-spoken, somewhat absent-minded scientist, has worked as an immunologist for more than twenty years. Like many scientists, he is at his most animated when talking about his own area of expertise, which in his case is the immune system: how it works, how cells interact, and—the main subject of his current research—biological response modifiers. Dr. Ghoneum received his undergraduate degree in zoology at Mansoura University in Egypt; did postgraduate work in histochemistry, radiobiology, physiology, and embryology; and began studying the immune system for his master's degree in 1973, also in Egypt. At twenty-six, he moved to Japan to work on his doctorate.

"My Ph.D. was on the effect of radiation on the immune system," Dr. Ghoneum explains. This made Japan, with its legacy of radiation in Hiroshima and Nagasaki, the natural choice. He did his postdoctorate at the UCLA School of Medicine, then moved to Drew University of Medicine and Science to head his own laboratory, carrying out National Institutes of Health (NIH) research on chemical carcinogens and their impact on the immune system. "For fourteen years," he says, "I worked on NIH grants [with my team] to study the effect of pollution on the immune system. The effect of inhaled chemical carcinogens from gasoline, cigarette smoke, car exhaust, and how this affects the immune system and cancer."

In 1991, during a workshop he had organized for a group of visiting Japanese immunologists, Dr. Ghoneum was approached by a very insistent Japanese gentleman who, through a translator, asked Dr. Ghoneum to "analyze" a substance that he had brought with him from Japan. Dr. Ghoneum gets such requests constantly.

He threw the packet in the wastebasket. "It's a lot of work to do a good analysis," he says, "and if I analyzed everything people wanted me to, I'd never get any work done." But the Japanese man was persistent, and, mostly to satisfy him, Dr. Ghoneum said he would do it. It would lead nowhere, and that would be that—or so he thought.

"I designed a simple experiment on mice," says Dr. Ghoneum now, "and the results were simply *amazing*." So amazing that he was sure he'd made a mistake. "I thought it had to be wrong. The induction of immune function in mice injected with this product was so significant, and so early, so quick," he says, "that within two days [there were remarkable changes] in the immune system."

Such a phenomenal result had to be an error; it simply didn't make sense. Just about any substance, any drug, requires time to work. Blood levels of the drug have to be raised enough to ensure that therapeutic quantities are coursing through the animal's system. It requires a minimum of a week to give the drug a chance to work. But the little packet from the insistent Japanese man had properties that were extraordinary—not only in terms of their effects but in terms of the speed with which these effects manifested themselves. So Dr. Ghoneum did the tests and assays again—with the same results. This, he decided, merited further study. By some accident of fate, this substance had landed in his lab. It was up to him now to discover what it was, how it worked, and how it might be used clinically.

### What Is MGN-3?

The chemical name of the substance that Dr. Ghoneum analyzed is *Arabinoxylan Compound*. Arabinoxylan occurs in grasses, such as rice shoots, wheat, and corn. It is the principal ingredient of *hemicellulose*, a kind of dietary fiber, which has been found useful for aiding gastric functions including absorption of nutrients and excretion of body wastes, and also for promoting growth of beneficial intestinal bacteria. It helps digestion, in other words. (The term *hemicellulose* is the general name used to describe a group of highly soluble molecular carbohydrates that resemble *cellulose,* the carbohydrate forming the skeleton of most plants.)

Arabinoxylan Compound, or MGN-3, is a patented blend of rice-bran hemicellulose B and shiitake mushroom. (Dr. Ghoneum slightly altered the original compound's chemistry.) It has been tested and found to be non-toxic.

What does MGN-3 do? Quite simply, it dramatically increases the activity of natural killer (NK) and killer (K) cells.

## The Immunomodulatory Effects of MGN-3

To discover the details about what MGN-3 was, how it worked, and at what dosage it would be most effective would require years of testing and research. Dr. Ghoneum is scathing about products on the market that haven't been tested scientifically and that are marketed with vague directions like "brew as a tea and drink." "A lot of people will say, 'Oh, I take this mushroom and boil it, 20 grams, and drink the soup.' How do you know it's 20 grams? How strong? Why not 2 grams? Why not 200? None of this has anything to do with science."

So Dr. Ghoneum began by testing various dosages using *in vivo* studies—studies on live subjects—with laboratory mice. To ensure that the animals' immune systems were depressed, he used his "own unique model for immune suppression: age—a phenomenon that cannot be argued with." With age comes a reduction in immune function—in laboratory mice and in other animals. To test the effect of MGN-3 on the immune system, Dr. Ghoneum used old mice with ailing immune-system function. He refuses to engage in what he calls "brutal" methods, like amputation or putting the mice under massive stress or exposing them to radiation. "When we get old, our immune system becomes poor," he says simply, "and we become prone to all sorts of diseases. So if you have old animals, not exposed to any external factors, merely age, this is associated with immune suppression."

Using one control group and one experimental group, he tested the substance MGN-3 again. Again, he got the same results: NK activity virtually tripled. "I dropped my work with the NIH, and since 1993 I've been working on this," he says. "I have done research and published articles on many areas related to immuno-suppression—aging, pollution, chemical carcinogens, stress." It seemed like a natural progression to go from understanding what could harm the immune system to experimenting with immune modulation and "how to push NK cells" to work better.

The next mystery was dose. Dr. Ghoneum divided rats into four groups, with five to seven animals in each group, to determine optimal dosage of MGN-3. He gave each experimental group a different dose, then measured each group's NK-cell activity after two weeks of putting MGN-3 in their food. The control group received only food.

"MGN-3 was found to be dose-dependent," writes Dr. Ghoneum in his research results. In the experimental group, NK activity was up 142 percent, 130 percent, and 119 percent compared with the control group, at daily doses of 50, 5, and 0.5 milligrams per kilogram of body weight, respectively. The effects were speedy, too: as early as four days post-treatment, particularly in the group given the highest dose (50 milligrams). Interestingly, the study also found that female rats responded better than the males—with an NK activity increase of 162 percent, compared with 135 percent for males (though what this sex difference might imply for humans is not clear).

In true scientific fashion ("each successful step leads to another," as he puts it), Dr. Ghoneum was ready to move on to *in vitro* studies, using human blood samples. "*In vitro*," he says, "you take someone's blood, separate the white blood cells from the red blood cells (since the NK cells are among the white blood cells), take the white blood cells and add the substance overnight. You also need a control, to see what would happen overnight without any intervention. The second day, you have the control, untreated, and the treated sample; add the cancer cell. Very simple experiment." The results continued to astonish him. An extraordinary number of the cancer cells in the experimental sample were destroyed, compared with those in the untreated sample.

According to the *immune surveillance theory,* it is the immune system—primarily the NK cells, when it comes to cancer—that should attack the cancer cell. But, says Dr. Ghoneum, only too often the opposite happens, and the cancer cell kills the white blood cell. "When the NK cell is weak, the cancer cell will extend its 'arm' around the white blood cell, fold its 'arm' around it, encircle it." The cancer cell then completely engulfs the white blood cell, which is still visible, or extends a cup-shaped pocket that wraps around the white blood cell.

"It's war," says Dr. Ghoneum. "If the immune system is strong, it can kill the cancer cell. But if the immune system is weak, then the cancer cell has its own weapons to destroy."

How can you tell whether the cell inside the cancer cell is indeed dead? Through the simple introduction of a blue dye. If a cell is alive, its membrane, or outer layer, is selective. It doesn't let anything in—not blue dye, not any useless substance. But if it's dead, then the membrane no longer can keep the cell intact; blue dye gets in and the cell turns blue.

To actually measure the action of MGN-3 when it is added to the mixture of white blood cells and cancer cells, the researcher must have some way of counting the number of dead cancer cells. It would be impossible to do this manually, so researchers add a radioactive material, chromium-51. Since dead cells will release radioactive materials through their nonfunctional membrane, the number of dead cancer cells will create a certain amount of radioactivity. This amount is measured with a gamma counter, which uses the amount of radiation to calculate how many cancer cells have been killed. "The more the radioactivity, the more cancer cells that have 'popped,' or been killed," says Dr. Ghoneum.

NK cells on their own, in the control sample, will kill a certain number of the cancer cells. "When we say that the NK activity is 35 percent," says Dr. Ghoneum, "what we mean is that after four hours the NK cells have killed 35 out of 100 cancer cells." With the addition of MGN-3, the NK cells double or triple their activity, killing that many more cancer cells. In other words, MGN-3 doesn't increase the *number* of NK cells but merely increases their potency; it's a "true" biological response modifier, which is defined as a nontoxic substance that has measurable effects on biological responses, such as those of the immune system.

Later on, in Part Four, we will examine in detail the way MGN-3 works in the body to fight cancer in living human beings. We will also look at the implications that MGN-3 may have for giving weakened immune systems the strength to fight invasions other than cancer. But first, we need to go back to the immune system itself to understand what happens when it goes haywire.

# Part Two

---

# Crossed Wires–
# When the Immune
# System Fails

# Chapter 6

# Allergies and Asthma

*"The deviation of man from the state in which he was originally placed by nature seems to have proved to him a prolific source of diseases."*

—Edward Jenner (1749–1823), English physician
and author of *An Inquiry into the Causes and
Effects of the Variolae Vaccinae, or Cow-Pox*

The immune system is not only idiosyncratic and individual, but changeable. Like a *Star Trek* shapeshifter, it changes form and function depending on its task and responds instantaneously to changes in the environment. It is the immune system's very complexity that also makes it prone to error—though comparatively few, given the number of reactions and interactions it makes within a single person's lifetime. But mistakes do happen. Think of it as being like airplane travel. Every minute of every day, hundreds of planes take off and land in airports all over the world, with hundreds of thousands of people on board. Most of the time, everything goes like clockwork: everything's on time, the baggage gets where it's supposed to; everyone arrives without incident. But now and then luggage does get lost, flights are late or canceled, and on occasion, there is a major disaster. Suddenly, the safety of flight seems in doubt as the news of a crash or a near-catastrophe unfolds on CNN.

Similarly, the immune system is prone to error largely due to the sheer complexity of its workings. It too has thousands of interconnections and a million details to contend with—and most of the time everything works just fine. But every so often, something goes wrong. Usually, it's nothing too terrible—the biological equivalent of lost luggage, a delayed flight, or a missed connection, like an allergy—but occasionally something goes spectacularly wrong. An individual gets struck with a debilitating autoimmune disease like lupus, or with a virus that leads to AIDS or cancer, or an immune-system reaction goes haywire, creating a fatal condition like encephalitis—or inflammation of the brain.

## IMMUNE MALFUNCTION

Simply put, the protective mechanisms of the immune system can go wrong in four basic ways. Sometimes, there is damage to the immune system through infectious agents or as a result of poisons or drugs (which may have been administered therapeutically—when someone is allergic to penicillin, for instance). In other cases, immune deficiency can come from general damage to the person as a whole, as can occur with malnutrition. In a small number of cases, the immune system malfunctions because of an inborn, genetic defect, the result of a flaw in the development of the cells responsible for immunity.[1] Some infants, for example, never develop a thymus and consequently are unable to produce mature T cells. Others are born with B cells that are unable to produce immunoglobulins. More commonly, what seems to happen is that through a combination of genes, environment, and overactive or underactive immunity, a normal reaction goes awry.

Often, as with allergies, the immune system seems to have become a little oversensitive—a touch hyper. But there are far more dangerous conditions that result from a normal immune reaction going awry, including life-threatening asthma episodes and fatal shock. Is there a connection between the increasing incidence of these conditions and the manipulation of the immune system through too much immunization? Perhaps.

## MISSED CONNECTIONS

To most of us, they're invisible, harmless little bits of pollen float-ing in the air around us. But to people with hay fever, they're the enemy. And if the millions of dollars spent on advertisements for antihistamines are any indication, all-out war has to be waged on the immune system in order to prevent the runny nose, watery eyes, sneezing, and other symptoms of hay fever and similar aller-gies.

In earlier chapters, we learned how the immune system reacts to what it perceives as a threat with two forms of immunity. Non-specific troops like macrophages and microphages, adaptive lym-phocytes like T and B cells and immunoglobulins, and all the attendant chemicals like interleukins and interferon rush in to pro-tect our integrity from any external threat. Within limits. When the immune response goes from being beneficial to harmful, the result is an *allergy* or *hypersensitivity*.

In ordinary conversation, the word allergy is used, rather loosely, to refer to any adverse reaction a person may have to a fairly ordinary substance, from a hand cream that causes a rash to a pet's hair that makes one sneeze. Immunologically speaking, however, an allergic reaction—it's also called *immediate hypersensi-tivity*—is an immune-system response. In other words, there has to be an identifiable immunologic reaction to something like dust or pollen for the reaction to be called an allergy. The substances that cause allergies were first called *allergens* in 1906, when they were first observed, since just like a serious threat (antigens), they trig-ger the immune system into fighting it off. Common allergens are pollens, certain drugs, lints, bacteria, some foods, dyes, and chem-icals.

*Hypersusceptibility*, in contrast, is a predisposition on the part of certain people to react to a chemical. For instance, people who say they're "allergic" to MSG, a food additive often used in Chinese cooking, are usually hypersusceptible to it. Exposed to sufficient quantities of MSG, most of us would have a reaction, but in the tiny amounts used in food to enhance flavor, it is usually not detectable. (There is, incidentally, no such thing as a "milk allergy." Some people simply lack the enzyme, lactase, that breaks down the lactose in milk. And this is rarely a long-term intolerance; most people can regenerate the enzyme if they gradually introduce milk into their diet. People without the enzyme can also take lactase tablets before eating a dairy-rich meal.) Then, there are some people with a genetically predisposed hypersusceptibility, which is called an *idiosyncrasy*. People who get migraines or hives from foods that rarely cause reactions—coconuts, for example—are displaying an idiosyncrasy.

## ALLERGIES

We've all seen people who start to sneeze when there's a cat in the same house. It's unclear why this happens to some people. After all, cat dander gets in everybody's nose. But only some people react. There does seem to be a genetic component, though, since children of parents with allergies are more prone to developing allergies of their own. Close to 50 million Americans currently suffer from allergies, and their numbers are on the rise.

There are four types of allergy: immediate, cytotoxic, immune-complex, and delayed. Immediate (also called Type I allergy) is the most common and involves the production of immunoglobulin E (IgE), one of the B-cell antibodies. People with allergies often have much higher levels of IgE in their blood than is normal. Unfortunately, this can't be used as a diagnostic tool because it is erratic. A person can have allergies without having detectable blood levels of IgE.

It is not the first time you're exposed to an allergen that you develop symptoms but the second, after the immune system's memory has kicked in. Much in the same way as vaccination creates a sort of "template" for the appropriate antibody, which can then quash a subsequent infection, an allergen first affects the immune system quietly. But once the substance has been identified, the second time it shows up your immune system launches a full-scale attack to flatten it with the IgE antibody. It's the immune system's response that creates the allergy symptoms, which can be in the respiratory tract (sneezing and runny nose), dermatological (hives or eczema), or gastrointestinal (bloating, diarrhea, and cramping).

The allergen goes in to rest on what are called *mast cells,* in one of the regions of the body where allergies are prone to occur. Mast cells are connective-tissue cells whose exact function is still somewhat mysterious. They function primarily through a chemical called histamine (hence *anti*histamine). Histamine plays an important role in the body's response to injury, particularly with respect to stress, inflammation, and allergies. It can make smooth muscles, like those of the lungs, contract, and it affects blood vessels. The mast cells that release histamine are particularly plentiful in the linings of the eyes, nose, lungs, and gastrointestinal tract, and are quite specific. In other words, once a mast cell develops IgE in reaction to cat dander, that same cell will not react to ragweed pollen.

Activation of the mast cells causes a variety of reactions, of which muscle constriction is one of the most common. These cells also cause relaxation of blood vessels in the skin—resulting in redness and irritation—or in the whole body, which can lead to the anaphylactic shock experienced by people who are allergic to bee stings. In some people, mast-cell reaction can cause edema—water retention—as the blood-vessel walls become more permeable, allowing fluid to build up in the tissues. There may be as many as 500,000 different and specific IgE antibodies on each mast cell's surface,[2] which explains why a person might be allergic to thousands of substances.

The allergic reaction, whatever form it takes, begins once the molecules of the allergen—dust, for instance—come into contact with the mast cell that is coated with the specific type of IgE "programmed" to react to dust. The presence of the allergen activates the IgE on the mast cell, which then releases chemicals with powerful inflammatory abilities. These include histamines, leukotrienes, and prostaglandins, as well as cytokines. This sort of reaction happens within moments of exposure to the allergen.

The other three types of allergy are rarer, slower, and often more serious. Cytotoxic hypersensitivity (Type II) comes on gradually, also after the person's second exposure to the allergen. This substance binds to the surfaces of blood cells to form a new antigen. Immunoglobulin G or M then binds to this new threat. The result can be an impairment of the blood-clotting mechanism, or anemia.

In immune-complex hypersensitivity—Type III allergy—a mix of IgG and other antibodies sits around in tissues, creating inflammation. If it ends up in the kidney, it results in an inflammatory injury to the kidney, glomerulonephritis; if it settles in the lung, it leads to a pneumonia-like condition. These two types of allergies do not seem to have a true allergic component—namely histamine—and the best defense against them seems to be simply avoiding the substance that triggers the allergy.

The fourth kind of allergy has a different mechanism altogether and doesn't have anything to do with B cells at all. Delayed hypersensitivity—Type IV allergy—involves T cells, which, in turn, cause inflammation. The inflammation can take the form of chronic pneumonitis in the lung or contact dermatitis on the skin. Symptoms of this type of allergy take anywhere from twelve to twenty-four hours to develop after exposure to the allergen. The time factor enables us to differentiate between Type IV allergy and an immediate, or Type I, allergy, which happens quickly, virtually right after contact. Contact dermatitis, for instance, occurs within minutes, if not seconds, after exposure to the allergen.

## LEVELS OF REACTION

It is not only the allergen but the site on the body that it affects that determines the kind of allergic reaction an individual will have. Allergic rhinitis, or hay fever, happens when pollen or another airborne substance to which the immune system has developed antibodies gets into the tissues of the nose. That's what leads to the quick, short sneezes, runny nose, and other discomforts experienced by hay-fever sufferers. Inflammation of the tissues also plays a part in the reaction. Similarly, allergic conjunctivitis affects the eyes when an allergen somehow gets into their fine linings. Although the skin is usually exempt from direct attack, in some people it can become allergic with eczema or atopic dermatitis after exposure to a substance to which the individual's immune system has become attuned—certain metals used in costume jewelry, for example.

## Inflammation

It was only recently realized that part of an allergic reaction is inflammation. Inflammation, which we discussed briefly in Chapter 2 (in reference to the acute-phase immune reactions that happen quickly in response to an injury like a cut or scrape), is a local reaction on the part of tissues, particularly the small blood vessels, to an injury or "physiological insult." Any process that damages tissue, whether it's infection with bacteria (or a virus), excessive heat or cold, or a physical assault on the tissues—a cut, a scrape, a bang, exposure to a harmful substance like acid—causes inflammation. At times, it is solely the inflammation that is responsible for whatever lack of function there may be—as in asthma, where it clogs up bronchial passages and prevents the sufferer from breathing.

## Asthma

A dramatic, violent, and potentially fatal reaction is *asthma*, a chronic lung disease that causes sufferers to cough, wheeze, experience tightness in their chests, and feel short of breath. It happens when inflammation causes a reversible obstruction of the airflow to the lungs. Although allergies are not the only cause of asthma, they are widely implicated in the beginnings of this debilitating and dangerous condition, which occurs in many Western countries in about 5 percent of people. The incidence of asthma has doubled in the past two decades. In the United States alone, more than 15 million people suffer from it.[3] It is the sixth most common reason for people—

especially children and teenagers—being hospitalized. Asthma-associated hospital expenses run in the billions ($6 billion in 1995), and each year more than 5,000 deaths are attributable to asthma attacks—a 111-percent increase since 1979.[4] African-Americans are three times as likely to die of asthma as other groups.[3]

The word asthma comes from a Greek word meaning "to breathe hard." People who suffer from asthma wheeze, gasp, and have episodes of being unable to breathe. Thick mucus comes out of their lungs when they cough. It's aggravated by stress, colds or chest infections, pollution, exercise, weather, certain drugs, dust, smoke, pollen, and other allergens in the air. People who have become sensitized to certain foods—common ones are shellfish, eggs, milk, wheat, peanuts, and other nuts—may have severe and even life-threatening symptoms after eating those foods again. Most complications from asthma arise from hyperresponsiveness, or oversensitivity, of the air passages, much of which is due to excessive inflammation.

A lesser, and less dangerous, form of asthma is exercise-related. It features the same wheezing and ripe coughing as the more serious kind, but it comes on as a result of strenuous exercise. Treatment consists of changing one's fitness regimen and learning to pace oneself, as well as some drug therapy.

Overall, there's been a dramatic shift in asthma treatment in recent years, away from symptom relief (using bronchodilators) to identifying the actual causes of airway reactivity and attempting to prevent that along with the inflammation. But even though treatments have become more sophisticated, the increase in the incidence of asthma is of great concern worldwide.

### Anaphylaxis

The most dangerous degree of allergic reaction is *anaphylactic shock,* which can be fatal if untreated. It causes inflammation and constriction of the air passages and is usually accompanied by an abrupt lowering of blood pressure, which can cause the heart to stop if adrenaline is not promptly administered. Adrenaline (or epinephrine) is a hormone secreted by the adrenal gland. It is instrumental in attention and memory, and it also stimulates the sympathetic nervous system to raise blood pressure, accelerate heart rate, and increase metabolism. It is responsible for the nervous feeling we may get when we are stressed, like stage fright. Excessive levels can be just as bad as levels that are too low.

The most common triggers of this dangerous allergic symptom are penicillin, stinging insects like wasps and bees, shellfish, peanuts, and latex—like that used in surgical gloves. Despite our growing body of knowledge about allergies and despite the many antihistamines available on the market, thousands of people die each year from anaphylactic shock caused by undiagnosed allergies. Fatal consequences can also be suffered by asthma sufferers who simply don't know they have asthma—their first major attack can be their last.

## A MEASLES CONNECTION?

There has been a dramatic increase in asthma as well as allergies throughout the developed world in the past few decades. This could be due to high levels of air pollution; to today's airtight, energy-efficient buildings, from which trapped poisons and chemicals can't escape; to increasing general ecological disturbance, which releases more pollens and other airborne allergens; or to the fact that many children were not breast-fed for some years after World War II.[5] But the most provocative explanation comes from a growing group of experts who believe that the increased incidence of asthma may have something to do with overzealous childhood immunizations aimed against too many childhood diseases— which makes sense, given that allergies and asthma are essentially immune-system reactions.

While agreeing that vaccinations play a vital role in preventing diseases—including polio and smallpox—that once killed most of the people they infected, these experts argue that perhaps routinely vaccinating children against too many diseases may be overkill. An example is the combination vaccine MMR, which immunizes children against measles, mumps, and rubella (also called German measles). Some British researchers have suggested that reducing the incidence of common childhood infections like measles may lie at the root of the rising incidence of asthma worldwide, and that it is not the environment but a faulty or inadequately developed immune system that we should hold responsible for the rising statistics.[5]

It is known that children who have measles are more infection-prone during that period of illness than usual. New research suggests that this may be due to reduced levels of interleukin-12, which is responsible for the "start-up" immune response to infection. This would seem to indicate that there is more going on during measles than solely a reaction to a virus—that the immune system is somehow fairly massively engaged. If that is so, then vaccinating children against measles might have untoward effects on the immune system in later life.

A British study that looked at asthma rates in nearly 30,000 children between 1973 and 1986 found that there were definitely higher rates of asthma among British children.[6] Further research suggests that, some of the time, the incidence of asthma decreased in proportion to common childhood diseases, measles in particular. In other words, children who'd had measles seemed to be less susceptible to asthma than children who had not. If it's indeed the case that the (usually) mild form of measles that children get has some impact on the developing immune system, then preventing it from happening through immunization might be detrimental in the long run. Intervening in the development of immunity through vaccinations might cause the immune system in later life to be oversensitive to normally harmless substances like ragweed pollen, animal dander, or grasses.

This concept makes a certain intuitive sense. As the immune system sails along without any early assaults, it does not incorporate into its workings the normal "checks and balances" that it should have. After all, we know that the immune system has a potent destructive force and that, were it unable to check its own reactions, it would end up killing our own cells.

Furthermore, we now know enough about the workings of the

immune system to realize that it reacts differently to an "artificial" form of a disease, as is introduced through vaccination, than to the natural infection. When natural infection occurs, certain helper T cells are called into play that are less likely to provoke an allergic reaction than those that react to a vaccine.[7] In a study done in the African country of Guinea-Bissau, it was found that young adults who had contracted measles as children showed less reaction to tests of allergic reactivity than those who had been vaccinated *and* those who had never had measles.[8] The authors write, "Epidemiological studies have led to speculation that infections in early childhood may prevent allergic sensitization but evidence to support this hypothesis is lacking. We investigated whether measles infection protects against the development of atopy (allergy) in children of Guinea-Bissau." Almost 300 young adults, first seen in 1978, 1979, and 1980, were followed up in 1994. Sure enough, it seemed that a natural bout of measles might well translate into protection against asthma and/or allergies. The authors also tested reactivity to allergens and found that 82 of 268 adults (31 percent) who'd had measles as children were *anergic,* or nonreactive to common allergens, compared with only 20 of 121 (17 percent) adults who had been vaccinated against measles.[9] The authors did not find that a natural bout of measles caused unexpected deaths—which is the rationale behind vaccinating against it in the first place.[10]

Nevertheless, measles can have severe complications, like deafness and brain damage. Issues such as the ones raised by these studies should not be taken as any sort of blanket statement that vaccinations are bad. Parents need to consult with physicians, nurses, and other health-care professionals to decide on the risks and benefits of vaccinating or not vaccinating their children. The point is that the safety of vaccines needs to be monitored and assessed on a regular basis: we can't afford to become complacent about the immune system.

## NATURAL PROTECTION

While the evidence is still inconclusive on the measles-asthma connection, there is a fair amount of anecdotal, or unscientific, evidence suggesting that asthmatic or allergic children who "grow out of it" may well do it through a bad natural bout of mumps or measles. One of the authors of this book had a serious case of eczema as an infant and young child that stubbornly remained resistant to all forms of therapy. By the time she was seven, large, itchy welts covered her legs, arms, and face. Then, at the age of eight, a bad case of rubella with a high fever wiped out every trace of the eczema. The general explanation at the time was that the dermatitis had been "burned away" by the fever that accompanied the infection, but it seems more reasonable, in the context of our present knowledge of the immune system, to say that the immune system became stimulated as a result of the rubella and managed to regulate its own reactions. The eczema, after all, was either an allergy or an autoimmune disorder, or a bit of both. The excessive sensitivity to normal stimulation went away, and the skin was no longer red, inflamed, and itchy.

We are not suggesting that vaccines should be thrown out the window. The process of keeping disease at bay is a fragile balancing act between keeping the integrity of the person intact and keeping "outsiders" out. But it may be that our internal "ecology" is just as fragile as the external environment about which we are finally becoming concerned. Just as the destruction of an Amazon rain forest or the holes in the ozone layer in the far north can have drastic and negative consequences for the weather in Houston or London or Shanghai, too much early manipulation of the immune system could backfire, with undesirable consequences in adulthood.

Similarly, our internal ecology seems to be subject to certain natural disasters—the physiological equivalent of earthquakes, tornadoes, and floods. When the immune system misreads a stimulus, the results can be what are known as autoimmune disorders—conditions in which the immune system turns on the host. These will be examined in the next chapter.

# Chapter 7

# Civil War—
# Autoimmune
# Disorders

*"To suffer in one's whole self is so great a violation, that it is not to be endured."*

—D. H. Lawrence (1885–1930), English writer

Think about those times you've been *really* rushed—and how much higher the odds are at such a time of making a silly mistake, having an accident, or otherwise getting things wrong. The same is true of the immune system. With its highly sophisticated and well-armed defense system on constant alert, there are times when it becomes overloaded and gets its wires crossed. Just like in a real war, the internal conflict against invaders can suffer from faulty intelligence or poor communications, or a rogue battalion might throw the soldiers off course—causing havoc and drastically affecting outcomes. Innocent bystanders can get hurt; even allies and friends can be destroyed. At times of high stress, when things become more complicated, even the decision-making process itself can become unbalanced.

Conversely, the immune system might take a course of action that is beneficial to one part of the organism but harmful to the whole. Sometimes, in war, to achieve one worthwhile objective it becomes necessary to sacrifice something else. During World War II, Allied forces allowed Coventry to be bombed so that the Germans would not realize their code had been cracked, and thousands of innocent civilians perished. So it is with the immune system at times. As it protects and defends the host, it must make decisions about which antigens, or invaders, to attack and which to let pass. Sometimes, in its zeal to repel an invader, immunity may end up doing more harm than good.

Autoimmune disorders are a frightening consequence of an overzealous immune system. In this chapter, we will explore these debilitating and sometimes fatal disorders.

## MONSTER CELLS

Take a fairly simple bacterium, like the one that causes tuberculosis (TB). It is not the *Mycobacterium tuberculosis* that is intrinsically harmful; rather, it is the aborted immune reaction to it that causes TB. When the bacterium first invades the body, it does so through the lungs. There, specialized macrophages recognize it as an invader and go on the offensive. Depending on the virulence of the bacterium and the strength of the macrophages, the bacterium will either be eaten or survive inside the macrophage, where there is a second line of defense, an "army" of enzymes that should manage to destroy it. But, should the TB bacterium manage to evade those enzymes, it then begins to divide and replicate itself *inside* the macrophage. Even then, it can remain relatively harmless, because this bacterium has a "waxy" coat that keeps it fairly separate from everything around it. Should the TB bacterium somehow be broken up, however, as happens in some cases, all hell breaks loose. The subsequent immune reaction creates cell and tissue damage far in excess of the original threat. This is called the *Koch phenomenon*, after the discoverer of the TB bacillus, Robert Koch (1843–1910), and refers to an immune-mediated reaction that is actually more harmful than the microorganism itself.

Most people with TB don't develop full-blown symptoms. In fact, only about 15 percent or fewer of those who get the disease actually become sick. Most at risk are children, the elderly, and those with compromised immune systems—like AIDS patients, many of whom develop TB. In most people, the macrophage simply holds onto the TB bacillus in a kind of "pathogenic détente."[1] It becomes a kind of monster cell, harboring the enemy. This can signal trouble.

Over time, these large mutant macrophages—and the resultant inflammation—release circulating cytokines, chemical messengers that act as a sort of clean-up crew for the immune-system war. The presence of cytokines, in turn, lets the T cells know that something is going on, and they come around to investigate. Like the crowd that gathers at the scene of an accident, the general chaos that eventually develops causes several of the TB-containing macrophages—the monster cells—to burst, releasing TB into the bloodstream. These TB fragments stimulate more macrophages, and the vicious cycle starts. The immune system sends in more troops, but the more involved it gets, the more TB-laden macrophages burst into the bloodstream. It's at this point that the patient starts to lose weight and to feel feverish, tired, and headachy and begins coughing up blood—all the symptoms of full-blown TB.

Eventually, if the TB bacillus is not "evicted," the T cells begin to wage war on the macrophages that are harboring it. The resulting chaos spills more TB out into the lungs, where the bacterium ends up skulking, chased by furious T cells intent on killing it. Now it's not just war, but carnage. Healthy lung tissue is destroyed, and whole segments of the lobes of the lung begin to almost liquefy. If antibiotics are not immediately given—and sometimes even if they are—the lungs give out, and the patient dies. Without a full-blown immune reaction, TB is not all that virulent. A quarter of the people infected with it don't get sick at all, and nearly half do not die of it, no doubt because the microorganism is "encased" in its little shell, and the immune system doesn't have to declare all-out war.

Similarly, autoimmune diseases are caused not by an external threat but by the immune system's turning on itself.

## HARDWARE FAILURE

It is the immune system's keen perception as well as its ability to distinguish the cells of the host (self) from that of an invader (not-self) that makes it all the more dangerous when it becomes excessively vigilant or somehow gets its wires crossed. It is, after all, a mechanism that's good at its job of destruction. And with all the different kinds of forces at its disposal—several kinds of T cells, B cells, natural killer cells, immunoglobulins, interleukins, interferon, and so on—when the immune system goes in with guns blazing, it's pretty effective. When it attacks the body's own cells, it does an equally good job. Lupus, scleroderma, Crohn's disease, multiple sclerosis, rheumatoid arthritis, Addison's disease . . . the list goes on, and so do the symptoms that sufferers experience.

For years, many immunologists simply could not believe that the immune system was capable of such treachery, even though Paul Ehrlich, one of the most brilliant scientists of the last century and a founder of the science that was to become immunology, did predict that it could happen. Ehrlich recognized that the distinction between self and not-self might be subverted in some instances, which he called a *horror autotoxicus*. It may have been Ehrlich's own bout with TB that convinced him of the awesome and destructive power of the immune system. In any case, later scientists didn't accept that this powerful "army," which was how the immune system was described, could possibly *cause* illness. For years, autoimmune diseases weren't classified in any scientific way but were thought to be aberrations or the result of some environmental trigger like a faulty therapeutic technique—for instance, a tainted blood transfusion.

Eventually, however, it had to be recognized that autoimmune diseases, in which the person's own immune system reacts with normal body components to produce disease or functional changes, do exist.[2] And many of them are truly nasty.

We still don't know very much about autoimmune diseases. The tendency to develop an autoimmune disorder does seem to run in families, indicating some genetic predisposition. Rather surprisingly from an evolutionary perspective, women of childbearing age seem more predisposed to them than men—which indicates a possible hormonal link. But exactly what goes wrong? It's hard to say. Several mechanisms of immune-system failure have been suggested. It's possible that chemical (drugs, additives, or other compounds), biological (like the TB bacterium), or physical (allergens) agents may damage or alter the components relating to "self" so that the lymphocytes no longer recognize them. Perhaps infectious agents "trick" the body into thinking they are not foreign (think World War II movies when Allied troops dressed as Germans to sabotage Nazi plans). It may be that the immune system goes haywire when some part of the body that's not normally exposed to circulating lymphocytes—like the lens of the eye—inadvertently comes into contact with them, triggering a response.[2]

What we do know is that, more often than not, these disorders are preceded by some kind of physiological or psychological insult. Then, once the immune system is engaged, it refuses to stop. It just keeps going, destroying normal tissue, overproducing scar tissue, and creating impediments to normal function. The "stop" or "off" signals that are normally activated when it's no longer appropriate to fight don't seem to work.

## HALT! WHAT'S THE PASSWORD?

As we saw in Chapter 3, cells recognize one another through a kind of identifying mark (we compared it to a bar code)—the major histocompatibility complex (MHC). (See the inset "MHC and Tissue Transplantation" on page 86.) In humans, this recognition factor develops very early, in the later stages of fetal development and in early infancy. Then, those cells with the appropriate MHC (which can recognize what tissues are "self") are kept on, while the others are destroyed or rendered inert.

There are two classes of MHC molecules. One type recognizes antigens inside a cell, and the other reacts to threats from the outside. People whose systems contain specific MHC markers—or

# MHC and
# Tissue Transplantation

*The fact that the major histocompatibility complex (MHC) develops so early in the life of the organism was shown in dramatic fashion by Brazil-born British zoologist Peter Medawar, who received the Nobel Prize for Physiology or Medicine in 1960.[1] Medawar—whose 1986 autobiography had the amazing title "Memoir of a Thinking Radish"—was the first to demonstrate that immunologic tolerance, or the ability to recognize "self," was present in fraternal cattle twins. These animals were similar in terms of what their immune systems considered "foreign," which led Medawar to theorize that while they were still developing in their mother's uterus, there was some trading back and forth of histocompatibility.*

*Later, by injecting white mice with cells from black mice, he showed that early exposure to "outsider" cells, during the developing stages of immunity, meant that the foreign cells would be accepted by the host. Medawar wrote: "This phenomenon is the exact inverse of 'actively acquired immune' [rejection] and we therefore propose to describe it as 'actively acquired tolerance.'"[2]*

*Medawar's notion had enormous implications for tissue transplantation: when we read that doctors are searching for a "good" or "close" match, what they're really saying is that they're looking for some level of histocompatibility. It also explains why the most effective donors can so often be close family members.*

*Interestingly, the immediate rejection of cells that are not our own can have therapeutic advantages. In bone marrow transplants given to people with leukemia, for instance, the transplanted bone marrow's attack on the recipient's bone marrow has positive consequences: it kills not only the bone marrow but the cancer as well. This is a clear indication that the immune system is programmed to keep itself free of "outside" influences; therefore any lymphocytes bent on attacking the "self" are eliminated, right from the start.*

identifiers—tend to overreact to certain kinds of antigens, which can be useful—or not. For instance, people with a specific kind of MHC marker are effective at fighting off viral infections and cancer—but they are also prone to some autoimmune disorders. Presumably, people who develop a bad case of TB are the ones whose MHC predisposes them to react to the bacterium. It must not be forgotten, however, that the general health of the host also plays a part. It's been well known for centuries that poor general health, poverty, and malnutrition put people at high risk for many infectious diseases.

Although we like to assign recognizable human characteristics to just about everything we describe, in medicine and elsewhere, the fact is that the immune system is not "aware" of what it's doing. Like a computer, which makes no conscious choices but simply does what it's been programmed to do, the immune system does not make moral or ethical choices about what antigens to "kill." It does what it is genetically programmed to do. It has no ability to discriminate or to "think" beyond that which was programmed into it in infancy. Of course, environmental triggers—stressors, chemicals, poisons—might alter it in some way, though details are still lacking.

Autoimmune disorders may not make intuitive sense in the grand scheme of things (why would our own immune system attack our own tissues?), but, says immunologist Mark Lappé in his book *Evolutionary Medicine* (1995), it may be the price we pay for having such a powerful disease-fighting mechanism in the first place.[3] "Why would a system that has evolved to protect the body have retained the capacity to engineer its destruction?" he asks. Well, it's a small price to pay for having survived through millennia in a world full of hostile microorganisms. Lappé says that even asthma might have had an evolutionary advantage—that an immediate immune-mediated constricting of the lungs might have kept them safe from harmful fungi. "As partial support for this novel theory," writes Lappé, "recent work has confirmed that about one in five asthmatics are allergic to spores of the fungus *Aspergillus,* an agent capable of producing a sometimes fatal lung disease known as aspergillosis." In its zeal to prevent this fungus from killing the host organism, the immune systems of some people may have become oversensitive to it.

So what happens to make the immune system interfere with its own workings or launch a direct attack on healthy tissues? It's impossible to say what happens in all autoimmune conditions, but through research into individual autoimmune diseases, we know that various immune mechanisms go haywire in different conditions. Over time, clues are adding up that are helping us decipher what may actually be happening. As often happens, though, treatment has lagged behind theory.

## SCLERODERMA AND
## SYSTEMIC LUPUS ERYTHEMATOSUS

Autoimmune disorders may involve a single organ of the body (as in thyroiditis, a disease of the thyroid gland, in the front of the neck) or many. Some involve only one type of tissue or substance in the body. Others are systemic—that is to say, their course runs throughout an entire system of the body, like the vascular system (blood vessels). One of the most invasive autoimmune diseases, which can attack virtually any organ in the entire body, is *scleroderma*. Systemic lupus erythematosus, usually referred to as *lupus*, is another in this spectrum of autoimmune diseases. These conditions are debilitating, make sufferers very sick indeed, and can have fatal consequences for many patients.

Scleroderma, also known as systemic sclerosis, is the most physically pervasive of them all. Fortunately, it is fairly rare, affecting about six in a million people. It involves the skin, arteries, kidneys, lungs, heart, gastrointestinal tract, and joints. Scleroderma usually begins with a strange whitening of the fingertips—often triggered by cold—called Raynaud's phenomenon, which can persist for many years with no other symptoms. Another early sign of scleroderma is an odd pattern in the fingernail. As the disease progresses, it begins to involve the skin, which first puffs up and then constricts, leading to a condition where patients feel as though their skin is literally "stuck" to their bones and muscles. The skin, especially of the face and fingers, becomes shiny, tight, and thickened. Puckering around the mouth gives the person suffering from scleroderma an odd mask-like look, and certain movements of the face and fingers become slow and difficult.

In some people, other parts of the body and other organs become involved, leading to difficulty in swallowing, shortness of breath, palpitations, high blood pressure, joint pain, and muscle stiffness and pain. Treatment consists mostly of symptom relief. Once the disease spreads to the kidneys and damages the lining of vital organs such as the heart, it usually has a poor prognosis: nearly half of all such sufferers die within five years.[4] Some are kept alive through dialysis and major interventions.

Although the exact reasons that people develop scleroderma are not known, there is some evidence that exposure to certain chemicals may bring it on in predisposed individuals. Inhaling or exposing the skin to solvents like trichloroethylene and exposure to vinyl chloride (now both banned substances) may be instrumental.[5] It has been suggested that silica, still used in some household products and in breast implants, may also contribute to the development of this disease.

What is known is that, for some reason, the person's own T cells become manic. Beyond that, the cytokines—perhaps interleukin-2—seem to push fibroblasts, which are responsible for creating scar tissue at the site of an injury, into overdrive. Under normal circumstances, when you've cut yourself or had an operation, your body's immediate reaction is to send over macrophages and lymphocytes that, in turn, stimulate cytokines and interleukin-1, interleukin-2, and interleukin-4. These stimulate the fibroblasts to create scar tissue and heal the wound—to create the "scaffolding" that's needed for repair. Then they leave. Stop. Halt. Get out. In scleroderma, they never seem to stop. They just keep on going, forming more and more tissue that then builds up around vessels, organs, and tissues. This presumably has something to do with the T cells and cytokines giving them the wrong "orders," since they are the generals in this particular army. Or it may be that fibroblasts, once they get past a certain point of activity, have an almost tumor-like ability to proliferate.

Given the complexity of the process, no doubt there are many other triggers involved, but basically, that's what an autoimmune disease is: a normal reaction gone wild. The result here is excessive and uncontrollable fibrosis (the creation of fiber) around vital organs and connective tissue.

The autoimmune disease lupus is considerably more common, affecting mostly adult women. It usually lets up during pregnancy and breastfeeding and then starts up again. Approximately six times as many women as men get lupus (some sources say that the figure is even higher).[6] It, too, involves agents of the immune system attacking connective tissue and surrounding body structures and eventually damaging them.

There are two forms of lupus. The systemic kind, which affects the body generally, is the more dangerous. Discoid lupus erythematosus (DLE) affects the skin, beginning with a rash that later scars. Systemic lupus erythematosus (SLE) also causes a rash, usually in a butterfly shape over the cheeks and nose, but it also makes sufferers weak, ill, and feverish, and causes joint pain, loss of appetite, nausea, and weight loss. Like scleroderma, it can cause problems in the heart, kidneys, or other vital organs as the connective tissue around them becomes fibrous and scarred. As with scleroderma, treatment is mainly directed at relieving symptoms; there is no cure.

Scleroderma and lupus are two of the most disabling autoimmune disorders, but there are many more. Rheumatoid arthritis, mixed connective tissue disease, retroperitoneal fibrosis, and polymyositis are some of the rheumatological ones, and there is evidence that antibodies, notably immunoglobulin G (IgG), are the factors involved.[7] Other autoimmune diseases can "attack" individual organs like the thyroid (Graves' disease, Hashimoto's thyroiditis), the adrenal glands (Addison's disease)—which, ironically, are normally supposed to control excessive immune-system activity—or the pancreas (diabetes). The gastrointestinal tract can be similarly affected—with Crohn's disease, or primary biliary cirrhosis, in the bile duct. Pernicious anemia targets cells in the stomach wall, and reactive disorders like juvenile-onset diabetes and arthritis, rheumatic fever, and Reiter's disease are set off by bacteria and then move to specific sites. It's impossible to comprehend the upheaval such a disease can create for patients, who often have no way of knowing at what pace their illness will progress but realize that, other than symptom relief, there is little medical science can do.

## COMING AT IT WRONG?

Some immunologists now suggest that perhaps the standard treatment for autoimmune disorders, which involves depressing the entire immune system—as is done for solid organ transplantation—may not be the best solution. To date, immune-system depression has not proven to be very effective, which may be because the real "cause" of the immune system's craziness is not being addressed. In some illnesses, where fibroblast production is the problem, perhaps it would make more sense to target those particular cells and their "bosses," the T cells, rather than the entire immune system. Some researchers even believe that we should actually consider *boosting* immune function. This group believes that excessive fibroblast growth, or excessive numbers of antibodies like IgG, is not an "accident"; that in certain individuals these cells are already programmed, or predisposed, to overproduction and need only a slight trigger to get going.[8] In other words, in some people, for unknown reasons, trigger-happy cells may be just waiting for the chance to rain fire on everything around them. If the immune system could be convinced to work "smarter," this might not happen.

Although there is no proof, per se, for this theory, the very lack of success medicine has had in treating these conditions would seem to indicate that a different paradigm, a different model, is called for in the treatment of autoimmune disease. As long as we hang on to our nineteenth-century notions of the immune system being solely a defensive system that's there to destroy invaders, we are impeded in our quest to find solutions to disorders of the immune system. The result is that we can't treat these conditions effectively; all we can do is control symptoms. That is not enough for the many people who have had their lives ruined by auto-immune diseases. In the United States, there are as many as 20 women in every 100,000 people who suffer from either lupus or multiple sclerosis (two diseases that strike women more often than men).[9]

An area that merits far more study than it has had is the role of psychological and emotional factors in autoimmunity. It has been well documented in recent years that many autoimmune diseases first appear after a person has had a trauma of some kind, physical or psychological. And individuals who suffer from these illnesses know that stress, fatigue, emotions, and moods play an enormous part in how they feel and how the disease appears to progress. But perhaps it has seemed contradictory to discuss stress or other psychogenic factors in the context of autoimmune disease—which is a result of an *overactive* immune system—since stress itself is an immune *suppressant*. Stress—what it is and how it affects the immune system—is explored in Chapter 8.

# Part Three

---

# The Environment
# and the
# Immune System

# Chapter 8

# The Hazards and Stresses of Modern Life

*"This is, I think, very much the Age of Anxiety, the age of the neurosis; because along with so much that weighs on our minds there is perhaps even more that grates on our nerves."*

—Louis Kronenberger (1904–), U.S. critic and writer

Stress is such a common concept in our lives that it's difficult to believe the term *stress* was coined only sixty years ago. Before that, if people were stressed, presumably they'd say they were anxious, or tired, or tetchy, or who-knows-what. In contrast, today we're keenly and routinely aware of the impact of stress on our lives, on our health, and on the development of illness. Stress, as it turns out, is implicated in everything from heart disease to multiple sclerosis, schizophrenia to eczema.

Simply put, stress is your body's nonspecific response to any demand placed upon it, whether physical or psychological. Anything that causes stress is called a stressor, whether it threatens, worries, upsets, speeds up, pushes, or motivates you. Stress is so often referred to as a negative thing that we forget that without stress, there would be nothing to react to at all—we'd be overcome by inertia. As Hans Selye (1907–1982), the Canadian doctor who "invented" the word *stress* (he took the term from physics, where it refers to any force or strain strong enough to deform something), once said: "Complete freedom from stress is death."

As a young researcher at McGill University in Montreal, Selye found that animals exposed to extreme cold, injections, and other stimuli all seemed to react the same way. First, they would adjust to whatever the stressor was; but if it continued, they would become ill. He then extended his work to include humans, studying their reactions to everything from emotional upsets to the flu.[1] His colleagues scoffed at Selye's work; at the time it seemed preposterous that so many different kinds of stimuli could lead to the same physiological reaction.

Now, of course, more than fifty years later, we are learning that stress of many kinds causes serious consequences, not just to quality of life but to health and sometimes to life itself.

## THE PHYSICAL IMPACT OF STRESS

Dr. Selye published his results in the journal *Nature* in 1935. There, he showed how stress was an adaptive response that, when excessive and prolonged, would eventually cause the adrenal glands to enlarge and the lymphatic system to atrophy, or degenerate, and could lead to disease and dysfunction. Repeated stress can even mimic AIDS: the animal or person can waste away, lose weight and hair, develop gastric problems, and succumb to infection. In mice, apparently, the stress response can even lead to a fatal condition called calciphylaxis, which causes calcium deposits throughout the skin and organs.[2] The thymus, the gland that T cells call home, can begin to shrivel after a lot of stress. This is direct evidence of the impact of stress on the immune system.

Under stress, *allostatic* systems in the body—that is, the parts of the nervous system that control heartbeat, blood pressure, and hormonal responses as well as the cardiovascular, metabolic, and immune systems—respond. If the stress does not let up, what seems to happen over time is that the physical events that constitute the responses to stress take on a life of their own and continue overresponding, even if the original stressor is gone. The chronic wear and tear of unresolved stress can therefore be considered physiologically as an "allostatic load." It can push susceptible individuals into chronic illness. Often, someone with a genetic predisposition toward a particular disease—such as diabetes or even schizophrenia—will develop it after a major stress, which suggests that if that stress had not occurred they might not have become ill, regardless of their genetic "map."

## INDIVIDUAL RESPONSES TO STRESS

It's practically a cliché these days to talk about the effect of stress on illness. When we become psychologically stressed as the result of an event—whether internal or external—how we respond is very much a factor of who we are. The stimulus, or the stressor, per se is not as important as the individual's reaction to it. Two people might react in completely different ways to the very same event, or stimulus.

Suppose two people get fired from their jobs. Mary Kay has been thinking for a long time about quitting her job and starting her own business. For her, losing her job is a positive thing, a way of making her entrepreneurial dreams come true. The change in her circumstances might make her feel slightly off balance for a while, but eventually, for her, getting fired will be a good and positive stimulus. Chris, on the other hand, has no desire to be his own boss. His work at Acme Conglomerate Life *was* his life. Furthermore, he was only a few years away from retirement. For him, being fired means not only a change in day-to-day activities, but fear (How will I make the mortgage payments?) and anxiety (Who will hire me at my age?). It's the *emphasis* we put on an event, the meaning we give to it, that makes it stressful, not the event itself— although it's generally accepted that certain major life events like divorce, marriage, the death of a close friend or family member, and serious injury or illness are stressful for everyone, albeit in differing degrees.

Another important point is that individuals differ in their

capacity to withstand stress and their ability to do well under pressure. We've all known people who thrive on racing around nonstop (one of the authors of this book is a prime example!) and whose schedules make the rest of us dizzy. Similarly, other people find even small amounts of stress difficult to handle. Selye himself was a hard-driving person who thrived on being busy and worked long hours. "There's a great deal of confusion about stress," he once said in an interview. "Stress is the body's nonspecific response to *any* demand placed on it, whether that demand is pleasant or not. Sitting in a dentist's chair is stressful, but so is exchanging a passionate kiss with a lover—after all, your pulse races, your breathing quickens, your heartbeat soars. And yet who in the world would forgo such a pleasurable pastime simply of the stress involved?! Our aim shouldn't be to completely avoid stress, which, at any rate, would be impossible, but to learn how to recognize our typical response to stress and then try to modulate our lives in accordance with it."[1]

A certain degree of stress, as has repeatedly been shown experimentally, is stimulating and improves performance (on exams, for example, where it was found that those students who were a little nervous but not panic-stricken did better than those who weren't anxious at all). Selye called good stress *eustress;* the prefix is the same one as in *eu*phoria and *eu*logy and means "good." It helps to think of the stress in our lives as a violin string. It has to have a certain amount of tension in order for the bow to be able to pass over it and make music. But if it is *too* tense, it snaps. The key is to keep one's *reactions* to stress at a manageable level.

Over the years, several techniques to control the stress response—from relaxation to cognitive-behavioral strategies, which teach you to control your reaction to a stressful event by putting it in a different context—have been developed and are increasingly accepted by both the general public and the medical establishment. Many people with heart disease, for instance, can actually help reduce their cholesterol level—in combination with diet and exercise and, occasionally, drug therapy—by learning to reduce anxiety and control the way they react to stressful events.

## IT'S ALL IN YOUR HEAD

One of the most extraordinary things about stress is that it is so completely a mental phenomenon. Suppose you are sitting alone, late at night, reading this book. Suddenly, you hear a noise and imagine there might be an intruder. Imagine, also, that in recent weeks there has been a mugger or rapist in your neighborhood for whom police are still searching. Your heart begins to race. Your pulse speeds up. Your palms feel sweaty. Then you realize it was the cat, or your teenager coming home. Suddenly, just as quickly as it began, your heartbeat slows, your pulse stops racing, and everything goes back to normal, and you laugh at your overactive imagination. But in those few seconds when your cerebral cortex was telling you that something potentially dangerous could happen, your limbic system—the part of your brain that is concerned with emotion—had already contacted your hypothalamus.

The hypothalamus is a tiny area, weighing less than four grams, in the top central part of your head. Dangling from it is the pituitary gland. (If you put your finger on the bridge of your nose, your finger will be only a few inches away from the pituitary gland.) This is "mission control" for hormone levels, water balance, food intake, sexual rhythms, and the autonomic nervous system, which governs involuntary actions. The hypothalamus is highly sensitive. The slightest touch on this small part of the brain during neurosurgery can send the patient's temperature soaring and even bring on a coma. The hypothalamus is also responsible for creating states like fatigue, hunger, anger, and calmness. It is, in short, the central command post for the physiological processes that are connected to your emotions.

Under stress, the rear region of the hypothalamus, which regulates mood, produces *adrenocorticotrophic hormone.* ACTH, as it is called, stimulates the pituitary gland, just below the hypothalamus, and the adrenal glands, a pair of small, triangular-shaped hormone-stimulating glands behind the kidneys. The adrenal glands are responsible for putting a stop to a full-blown immune reaction—which, if left unchecked, can lead to an autoimmune disease. (These, incidentally, are the glands that malfunction in Addison's disease, a rare autoimmune disorder that afflicted both former President John F. Kennedy and the British writer Jane Austen—though by JFK's time it was treatable.)

In response to this message from the hypothalamus, the adrenal glands charge up their production of two hormones: adrenaline and noradrenaline. These create the famous "flight (noradrenaline) or fight (adrenaline)" response. Other hormones released into the system include endorphins and dopamine—which, among other things, affect pain perception. These hormones are the reason that soldiers in the heat of battle often don't feel even the most grisly wounds, but the same men will feel pain from a far less serious injury during peacetime or in the hospital. The chain of events started by the hypothalamus also includes the production of *cortisol,* one of the so-called glucocorticoid hormones, which immediately boosts the number of quick-acting phagocytes—the "eating" white blood cells—and reduces the circulating lymphocytes and macrophages.[3] In addition, oxygen and nutrients are sent to organs that might need them. Selye called this the "general adaptation syndrome."

The importance of this process to the immune system has been shown in experiments with laboratory rats: when their hypothalamus is destroyed, their immune function is drastically reduced.[4]

## STRESS AND IMMUNITY

For years there have been unscientific reports that stress can affect the immune system and increase vulnerability to illness and infection, and in recent years science has backed up this claim. A California study of 236 preschoolers found that the children who responded to stress with elevated blood pressure did indeed get sick more often.[5] The same researchers also found that kindergarten children who were stressed at having to go to school—whose immune-reaction function was measured through the level of corticol they secreted in their saliva—did, in fact, experience changes in their ability to make antibodies. Interestingly, the children who reacted strongly to stress coped *better* than their peers with low-stress events. That finding would explain why moderate, regular exercise, which is a slight stressor, seems to be of such benefit immunologically, while *too much* exercise depresses the immune system.

It seems to be cortisol, the main stress hormone, that does the most to negatively affect immune-system function. Cortisol is similar chemically to the corticosteroid drugs given to depress the immune system after transplants and to treat autoimmune disorders, and it affects lymphocytes, macrophages, and leukocytes and depresses certain cytokines like interleukin-2. When there is a lot of cortisol in one's system, otherwise active lymphocytes don't respond as well to various "threats," and the inflammation response is subdued. Oxygen-rich blood tends to be reserved for areas that might need "repair" during a crisis, and non-essential functions like digestion are ignored—which might explain why people often experience stomach problems when they are stressed.

But how does the brain—technically, the neurons of the brain—interact with the cells of the immune system? That was the question until 1980, when neuroscientist Candace Pert, Ph.D., then chief of the brain biochemistry branch of the National Institute of Mental Health, discovered *neuropeptides*.[6] These are brain chemicals that seem to act as "messengers" between the mind and the immune system. Certain white blood cells in the immune system have receptors that fit neuropeptides exactly, in much the same way that antibodies and antigens create a key-and-lock fit. What keeps the system balanced are the messages going *back* to the brain from the immune system, in the form of the ever-present cytokines that signal back "message received" and thereby prevent more hormones from being released.

The discovery and exploration of neuropeptides opened up a new field of study: psychoneuroimmunology, or PNI for short, which looks at the mind-body interaction and its effects on disease. Other evidence of the brain-body connection includes the presence of nerve endings in various immune organs like the lymph nodes and spleen, nerve endings that seem to be essential to the normal workings of the immune system. If the spinal cord—where those nerves originate—is damaged, the consequences can be terrible. Mice that have had their sympathetic nervous system compromised as a result of spinal damage develop autoimmune diseases, and normal functions, such as metabolism, are disrupted.[7]

There's also some connection between endorphins, our body's naturally produced painkillers, and natural killer (NK) cells. When lab rats are subjected to random, sudden electric shocks, their NK-cell count goes down. That suggests that the cortisol levels brought on by stress may play a central role in tumors and viral infections. Old rats exposed to stress have a "marked inhibition" in the capacity of their NK cells to bind to tumors. Furthermore, their lymphocytes appear to redistribute between different tissues.[8] Mice stressed through physical restraint have been found to make antibodies, but their cellular immunity plummets—so their ability to ward off viral infections is lowered. In addition, a recent study of women with cancer (a major stress!) has shown that killer (K) cell activity was severely reduced in those women who reported feeling most overwhelmed, stressed, and anxious.[9]

Other studies have shown that support groups and emotional backup seem to help cancer patients. An often-cited study done by David Spiegel of Stanford University, for instance, found that women with breast cancer who attended support groups lived nearly twice as long as those who did not (37 months compared with 19). "Believe me," Spiegel was quoted as saying at the time, "if we'd seen these results with a new drug it would be in every cancer hospital in the country."

There is also some connection, though it is poorly understood, between depression and physical illness. Some of it is probably due to the vicious cycle of illness, which causes depression, which then makes the disease worse, and so on; but there is evidence that mood itself has an impact on illness. For instance, it's been shown that antidepressants can increase NK-cell counts in cancer patients, which would seem to indicate that even a major disease such as cancer is affected by your emotional state.[10]

## FEELINGS AND THE IMMUNE SYSTEM

More than three decades ago, Dr. George Solomon, a Stanford University physician, wrote an article called "Emotions, Immunity and Disease: A Speculative Theoretical Integration." He had become interested in the subject when he realized that his patients with rheumatoid arthritis (RA, remember, is an autoimmune disorder) seemed to suffer more flare-ups of their disease during difficult times in their lives. Today, he could cross out the word "speculative"; what we've learned in the meantime about the immune system and how it's affected by emotions, thoughts, coping strategies, and general attitudes has filled many more articles and a lot of books.

Dr. Solomon noted some interesting similarities between our psychological "systems" and our immune systems. For instance, they both remember previous events, they are both adaptive, and both work to defend the organism—the self. The immune system defends us against microorganisms, and the mind defends us against pain, stress, information overload, and so on. Furthermore, writes Henry Dreher in *The Immune Power Personality*, inadequate or inappropriate defenses in either case lead to vulnerabilty to illness.[11] And with both systems, a previous exposure to a "toxic" stimulus can lead to either tolerance or extreme sensitivity. An extreme emotional trauma early in life, like the loss of a parent, either can be a source of inner strength or can mean that fear of future losses becomes an ever-present source of pain. By the same token, the immune system can shore up its defenses upon meeting a pathogen (as it does with vaccination), or become ultra-sensitive to it (as in allergies). Another similarity between the two systems is that they cannot function without an ability to communicate.

Spurred by this research, others took up the banner and, over time, showed how even rats could be taught to control an autoimmune disorder (lupus) through *biofeedback*—which is, in essence, learning how to "read" your own physiological processes, like heartbeat or increased T cells. Other researchers showed that it was impossible to predict illness on the basis of how much stress a person had experienced in his or her life. Instead, it was one's "faulty" *reactions* to stress that were instrumental in creating disease. Interestingly, it is not getting angry or having negative emotions that causes stress-related problems and illness; rather, it is the suppression of those feelings that's harmful. "Deadening" our feelings and repressing our emotions seem to have a toxic effect. So Woody Allen may not have been far wrong when he said: "One of my problems is that I internalize everything. I can't express anger; I grow a tumor instead."

Laughter—joy, mirth, humor—is another area that is just starting to interest researchers. Results are still preliminary, but it does appear that the way people habitually deal with their lives, whether cheerfully or negatively, affects their health. One Japanese study even suggests that laughter may have an impact on NK and other white blood cells.[12] "Laughing [appears to] increase the NK activity of people whose activity levels are below average and normalizes the CD4/8 ratios of people whose ratios are above or below the standard levels," write the authors. That implies that laughter has a kind of normalizing effect on both our moods and our immune system.

## EXTERNAL STRESSORS

Stress has another, lesser-known connection to illness—and it's nothing to laugh about. Stress increases a person's sensitivity and reactivity to toxic chemicals. When birds, for example, are stressed by eating 10 percent less food than normal, their ability to process the pesticide DDT is sharply lowered.[13] That tells us that stress plus chemical pollutants can translate into a deadly duo.

Life has always had its hazards, and there's little question that in terms of comfort, ease of everyday life, longevity, and health we live in a time that is unparalleled for its benefits. Throughout most of history, people were far more concerned with the ravages of typhoid, smallpox, diphtheria, and other diseases than they were about stress. Nevertheless, in the past twenty years North American life has become much more complicated. One poll estimates that the average American had twenty-six hours of leisure time per week in 1973, compared with fewer than seventeen hours today.[14] During the same period, the time devoted to doing chores, chauffeuring children around, and commuting has ballooned from an average of forty-one hours per week to more than fifty. According to various estimates, between 50 percent and 70 percent of doctor visits are stress-related. While undeniably difficult for the individual, these statistics have a more insidious side: how does our level of stress affect our physical reactions to the multitude of toxins that are in the food we eat, the air we breathe, and elsewhere in our comfortable modern society? Everyday substances from dry-cleaning fluids to insect spray contain toxins of one kind or another. Too much stress can increase our susceptibility to these poisons, just as the birds' susceptibility to DDT was increased.

## THE STRAINS OF MODERNITY

Although the terms and metaphors we use to describe immune functions have their roots in the work of Metchnikoff, Pasteur, and other nineteenth-century thinkers, we live in a very different world. At the turn of century, the leading causes of death were pneumonia, influenza, and tuberculosis. Today, the killers are heart disease and cancer. As the Swiss medical historian Henry E. Sigerist (1891–1957) wrote some forty years ago, "The development of industry has created many new sources of danger. [But while] occupational diseases are socially different from other diseases, they are not different biologically."[15]

Since Victorian times, spurred by the rapid growth of technology, external stressors such as chemicals and pollutants have increased dramatically. Everywhere we look—at our workplaces, in our homes, on our vegetables, even in our meat—there are chemicals with the potential to damage the immune system. Between 1942 and 1962, pesticides, insecticides, and fungicides were thought of as a kind of panacea, a solution to the problem of the many tiny creatures and microorganisms plaguing humanity, destroying crops, and spreading disease. What was not foreseen was the extent to which the targets of this biological warfare would adapt to the new threat—or the extent to which the substances would penetrate into the foods they were supposed to protect. In 1962, biologist Rachel Carson, in her extraordinary book *Silent Spring*, warned of the havoc to which these practices could lead. She was ridiculed. This was the age of newer and better technologies that were going to make America great. How could there be a downside?

But a downside there was, and the worst part of it is the longevity and wide-ranging scope of those pesticides. They turn up everywhere, found in dead whales in the Arctic and mutant frogs in Costa Rica. In June 1998, the United Nations met to discuss the ongoing problems of DDT and other toxins, many of which are banned in the United States but still widely used in many parts of the world. (In central Africa, for instance, DDT is used to control malaria, which is passed to humans via infected mosquitos.)[16] Twelve chemicals, including dioxins, PCBs, and other industrial compounds, have been found to play a role in birth defects and cancer as well as ecological disruption. The news continues to report on the residual effects of industrial waste once commonly dumped in rivers and landfills, from Love Canal in Niagara Falls to Minamata Island in Japan—the site of widespread and debilitating mercury poisoning from the sprawling Chisso plant.

Less newsworthy but even more insidious are the day-to-day effects and stresses we experience—sometimes resulting from supposedly benign workplace chemicals. A study of 289 individuals exposed to different chemicals in a computer manufacturing plant—generally thought of as one of the cleaner industries—displayed massive immune abnormalities.[17] Dr. Mamdooh Ghoneum, one of the authors of the study and the researcher working on MGN-3, for over a decade carried out research on chemicals and toxins and their effects on the immune system. He has found that exposure to even small amounts of many common chemicals, including benzene, asbestos, benzidine, and resins, not only increases susceptibility to cancer, as is well known, but can also cause autoimmune and other disorders.

"For many years, traditional methods for toxicological assessment have implicated the immune system as a frequent target organ of toxic insult," writes Dr. Ghoneum, "following chronic or sub-chronic exposure to certain chemicals. [These cause] multiple immune derangement [including] decreased cell-mediated immunity, lymphokine production, natural killer (NK) cell function, and mitogen-induced lymphocyte blastogenesis."[17] Paradoxically, toxins can also make B cells hyperactive, which then causes many of the substances implicated in autoimmune disorders to increase. In computer-factory workers, for instance, markers of "autoimmune conditions including rheumatoid factor, anti-nucleic acid antibodies, IgG, IgM, and IgA immune complexes and myelin basic protein antibodies (thought to be instrumental in causing multiple sclerosis) were clearly demonstrated." Those dry words conceal a frightening immune picture that results from the "comforts" of modern life.

There is another difference between our world today and that of the immunology pioneers, and that is the greatest threat to the immune system that medical science has yet discovered. It's AIDS, of course—acquired immunodeficiency syndrome—a disease that renders formerly healthy people as immunologically fragile as David, the Bubble Boy. In the next chapter, we will look at what happens when a virus renders the immune system powerless.

# Chapter 9

# AIDS—Immunity Under Siege

*"Acquired immune deficiency syndrome—AIDS—is both literally and metaphorically the cancer that can be caught. It is the penultimate surrender of the ill to the illness, an involuntary succumbing, a giving up. The invisible hostility of the world becomes visible, palpable, apocalyptic."*

—Sallie Tisdale, U.S. nurse and writer, *The Sorcerer's Apprentice: Medical Miracles and Other Disasters* (1988)

No other disease in history has resonated with the same religious, moral, and political overtones as AIDS—and no other virus has ever wielded the same grisly power over its victims. Human immunodeficiency virus (HIV) and AIDS have struck at the very heart of medicine and its core belief: that to cure disease, it is enough to eradicate the cause. Here, the cause is the immune system itself, since once HIV has staked its claim, one's own cells turn traitor. And the victims of AIDS are those usually least prone to illness: young, healthy men. Like a speeding train, AIDS derails its victims, then weakens them and makes them susceptible to infections that were seldom seen before—like Kaposi's sarcoma, a rare form of skin cancer, and *Pneumocystis carinii* pneumonia (PCP), another uncommon condition.

It is AIDS that has been responsible for focusing long-overdue attention on the importance and the role of the immune system in health and disease. And because it not only engages but subverts the immune system, AIDS is a promising arena for research into *immunotherapy*—treatment processes that work through modulating the immune system. That alone makes it important to understand how HIV behaves once it gets a foothold in the body.

## HOW AIDS BEGAN

Over the years, there's been much speculation and controversy about how AIDS started. According to the newsmagazine *The Economist*, "Popular conspiracy theories include the idea that it escaped from a military laboratory in the country of your choice or that it is part of a western racist plot to reduce the population of Africa, and there has even been a suggestion that it piggy-backed around on an early polio vaccine." The most popular idea about the spread of AIDS to North America was that a homosexual flight attendant brought it here. But with the recent discovery of a blood sample given to some American doctors in 1959 in the Congo, this speculation can be laid to rest.

The origins of AIDS lie in the near past, some time in the late 1950s or early 1960s, in Africa. Someone—nobody knows who—in what was then called Zaire (now the Democratic Republic of Congo) tangled with a chimpanzee. This person came away with more than he bargained for: the human version of SIV, or simian immunodeficiency virus, a virus formerly known only in monkeys.[1] Had this unknown person, "patient zero," simply gone on to die quietly, HIV, the human equivalent of SIV, would have disappeared off the face of the earth. Unfortunately, right around that time, Zaire exploded into one of the bloodiest civil wars in African history. War—and its attendant unsanitary conditions, refugee camps, and general mayhem—is the ideal breeding ground for any disease, from typhoid to the plague, and AIDS proved no exception. The disease spread and within a decade had begun to make waves in the developed world, in places like the United States. So "patient zero" was not the flight attendant but an anonymous resident of Africa. As to exactly how it happened, we just don't know and probably never will.

What we do know is that HIV comes in a number of different strains. The African virus is known as HIV-1, a fast-moving virus that subdivides into other strains with deadly speed. (HIV-2 came from the sooty mangabey monkey, or so it is believed.) Had HIV-1 not been such a fast microorganism, it might never have spread as quickly as it did across the continents.

**IMMUNITY UNDER SIEGE**

Before AIDS began its deadly odyssey, the importance of the immune system for health and a well-functioning body had been understood, but more in an abstract sense than at any realistic level. With AIDS, however, the medical community realized that a virus that attacks the immune system causes, in very short order, disease, disability, and death. Suddenly and dramatically, it became obvious just how essential the immune system really is. Terms like *cellular immunity* and *T cells* hit the front pages.

As researchers struggled to understand just what happened to the immune system with HIV, people took to the streets demanding action. Because HIV is transmitted through body fluids—blood and semen, primarily—it was first a disease of young homosexual men and intravenous drug users. Unfortunately, over time, people with hemophilia and others who'd received blood transfusions, babies, and other "innocents" who'd never had anything to do with unsafe sexual practices or drugs began getting the disease as well. Today, AIDS is rapidly reaching "epidemic" proportions. In 1997, the number of people infected with AIDS worldwide was 5.6 million.[2]

"Stopping the epidemic is of paramount importance," warned *The Economist* in July 1998. "AIDS is expected to come fifth on the World Health Organization's list of global causes of death by the end of this year (2.3 million people died of it in 1997). By the middle of the next decade, it will probably be third. At the beginning of 1998, more than 30 million people—about 0.5 percent of the earth's population—were infected with HIV, even though most of them had not yet developed the symptoms of AIDS. That figure has grown by a third in the past two years." Alarmingly, it is in the poorer nations of Africa that the disease has progressed most quickly. In parts of Botswana and Zimbabwe, one quarter of the adult population is infected. AIDS is now creeping into formerly AIDS-free zones such as eastern Europe as well, where rates of infection have increased seven times over the past three years. The same is true in China.

In the United States, the toll is well over half a million. Although homosexual and bisexual men account for fewer than half of new cases, they still represent the largest single group of AIDS patients. Intravenous (IV) drug users make up the next-largest group: of 74,000 new cases of AIDS reported in 1995, 35 percent were associated with IV drug use. The Centers for Disease Control and Prevention (CDC) estimate that HIV is the leading cause of death among men between the ages of twenty-five and forty-four and the third most frequent cause of death among women in the same age group.[3] A disproportionately high number of African-Americans die from AIDS: the death rate is nearly four times as high for black men as for white men (and nine times as high for black women as for white women).[4]

## HOW AIDS DEVELOPS

It's not possible to do justice to a subject as complex as AIDS and its effects on the immune system in one short chapter. Here, however, is a brief overview of what we know (or think we know) about AIDS and its precursor, HIV, which most—though not all—scientists believe is the cause.

HIV is what's called a *retrovirus*. Retroviruses are a specific class of virus that don't carry their own DNA; they have its sister compound, RNA, instead. In order to multiply, they need to attach themselves to a host and use the host's DNA to propagate. So when HIV enters the bloodstream, it must first invade a cell and take over its DNA.

Think back to Chapter 3, where you first made the acquaintance of helper and suppressor T cells. These T cells react to antigens, or foreign invaders, on the basis of their MHC markers—the "bar codes" of the antigens—which are called Class I and Class II. The T cells that attack Class I MHC antigens are known as CD8 cells, and the ones that attack Class II MHC antigens are called CD4 cells. It is the number of CD4 cells that determines whether a person has enough immunologic strength to fight off infection— that gives an indication of whether the immune system has its fighting strength. Most experts believe that HIV's favored target is the CD4 cell; though, according to another theory, HIV actually disrupts the production of cytokines (those same scavenging "halt" cells that play a role in autoimmune disorders). Yet another theory suggests that HIV kills immune function by inducing "autoantibodies" or by stimulating T cells in a way that causes them to self-destruct.[5]

The fact that there are so many conflicting theories makes it clear that we still don't really know what the exact mechanism is— or if it differs in different people and for different types of HIV. Nevertheless, the identifying mark of AIDS is the CD4 cell population. As the disease progresses, their number drops dramatically. A person sick with AIDS can lose most of these cells—leading, predictably, to profound immune deficiency. "One clue to the rapidity of this decline is the immune status of the host at the time when the HIV first takes hold," writes Mark Lappé in *The Tao of Immunology.* "If the body is already in a state of immunological overdrive, say as a result of concurrent sexually transmitted disease (STD) or a malarial parasite infection, HIV finds [more] receptive cells much more quickly [which] makes AIDS a much more deadly disease in Africa where parasites are rife." In other words, if the person's immune system is already forming antibodies in response to something else, and HIV comes along, that person is far more likely to succumb. This makes sense—and is true of most viruses.

Although the general feeling in the scientific community is that HIV directly kills cells, there is compelling evidence to suggest that there is more going on than a simple "war" on the immune system. It's been known for more than thirty years, for example, that *any* retrovirus can cause immunosuppression,[6] in which case both cellular immunity and humoral immunity become depressed as the body responds to the virus. By extension, then, the drugs that have been found to slow the progression of HIV by preventing it from replicating in the CD4 cell (through preventing the conversion of RNA into DNA[7] and therefore the ability of HIV to reproduce itself) may actually work by preventing the resultant immunosuppression rather than by reducing the amount of HIV in the blood.

Whatever the mechanisms of the actual disease process, what happens with the virus is reasonably straightforward. HIV enters the CD4 cell, sheds its protective protein coat and releases RNA, transcribes DNA from RNA, and then makes copies of itself. This, in effect, destroys the CD4 cell—which is now, for all intents and purposes, HIV. Then, as new viruses are formed (and as HIV multiplies), they move into the body to infect susceptible lymphocytes in the bloodstream. Soon the viruses enter the bone marrow itself. Some researchers believe that, along with the virus, this process so "warps" the CD4 cells that they become "foreign" to the body—they take on such a good disguise that they fool the immune system itself—and that these mutated CD4 cells are then attacked by other immune cells, notably CD8 cells, which could signal the beginning of full-blown AIDS.

The severity of HIV infection is determined by either measuring CD4 cell counts or measuring the amount of HIV in the body. A decrease in CD4 or an increase in viral load means that the disease is progressing. Until recently, efforts to measure the amount, or *titer*, of HIV in the blood relied on insensitive techniques that required being able to "grow" HIV in the laboratory. These were useful enough for research but were completely ineffective clinically. In the last couple of years, however, it's become possible to measure the relationship between the number of circulating virus particles and the rate at which AIDS develops. This is done through detecting the virus's RNA in blood. The titer of circulating virus is called the *viral load*. Several different groups of researchers have demonstrated that the HIV RNA in plasma (the fluid portion of blood) is directly proportional to the stage of the disease: high titers, between 100,000 and 1 million, occur initially, but once the immune system kicks in they can go down as low as 10,000.[8] Eventually, HIV depletes the CD4 cells. That leads to immunodeficiency and the various opportunistic illnesses that strike AIDS patients, who literally waste away.

## AIDS SYMPTOMS

Early HIV symptoms are nonspecific and difficult to spot, making early intervention difficult. They resemble the symptoms of infectious mononucleosis or a bad flu: swollen lymph nodes, headache, fever, fatigue, stomach problems, weight loss. As with anything else, any concurrent existing condition makes one more susceptible; so does one's genetic background. Individuals differ in their immune system "markers," as we saw in earlier chapters, and those with certain kinds of human leukocyte group A (HLA) antigens—involved in the MHC that identifies your molecules as "self"—seem more resistant to AIDS. It is thought that certain kinds of HLA create a strong initial immune response to HIV, whereas other types of HLA fail to bind to the virus and allow it to rage unchecked throughout the body.[9]

Over time, as the immune system becomes more "crippled," AIDS patients begin to fall prey to other, opportunistic infections. In the West, the infections are often pneumonia, yeast (fungal) infections, Kaposi's sarcoma, and mental symptoms (AIDS dementia complex) that develop as various organisms attack tissues of the brain. In Africa, tuberculosis and malaria are usually the diseases that AIDS patients succumb to. Without an effective immune system, the person is vulnerable to just about any viral or bacterial infection, and it is usually these that kill the patient rather than HIV/AIDS itself.

Although there are a number of very expensive drugs that appear to control AIDS in some people, many experts feel that the immune system should be engaged more in the fight against AIDS.

"We have not yet begun to tap into the potential of the immune system," said one doctor speaking at the Canadian Conference on HIV/AIDS Research in Quebec City in 1998.[10] There are people infected with HIV who don't seem to get sick with AIDS—or have not to date—and these patients are of huge interest to researchers. In some cases, early detection of the virus and immediate therapy seem to "kick start" the immune system into mounting its own defense. But this area of intervention is still in its infancy.

## PREVENTING AIDS

Although genuine public-health prevention measures, when undertaken well, can and do have an impact on the spread of AIDS, this is one disease to which politicians have been reluctant to react in traditional ways. Perhaps because AIDS is so associated with sex and drugs, many officials have not had the political will to put money into public education programs on prevention. The general fear seems to be that teaching people to take precautions, like using condoms or providing needle-exchange programs, implies approval of certain lifestyles. Yet, when public information measures have been put into place, their success rate has been phenomenal. One CDC official estimates that the United States' AIDS prevention budget (a little over $600 million) would need to prevent only 4,000 cases a year to pay for itself.[10]

Senegal, a country of western Africa, has had one of the world's most successful anti-AIDS campaigns. Reacting swiftly to the AIDS threat more than a decade ago, the country's predominantly Islamic and secondarily Catholic clergy were asked for their support right from the start, and their participation was invaluable. Sex education in schools was made mandatory, and there was heavy "social marketing" of condoms. People at high risk for contracting AIDS, such as prostitutes and their clients, were targeted for educational efforts. And the government drove home the point with the one group of young men over whom it had total control: the army. The campaign appears to have changed the behavior of Senegalese youth, and the country's rate of HIV infection has remained less than 2 percent—compared to 13 percent in neighboring countries.

The idea of preventing AIDS through a vaccine has been around for some time. More than a dozen hopeful tries have been made at immunization. Only one, AIDSVAX, made by a small American firm, has gone on to be approved for large-scale trials (to find out if it really works). But there are major difficulties in making an AIDS vaccine. For one thing, the antibody response—the one stimulated by most vaccines—is rarely potent enough to get rid of HIV proper, so how likely is it that a watered-down version will be effective? Too, since HIV appears to directly attack T cells (the CD4 cell), the vaccine would do so also, leading to full-blown AIDS. Furthermore, exactly what to use in a vaccine is a controversial issue. Some researchers believe that fragments of several proteins from inside the virus should be used, while others think it should be the protein that coats HIV. Still others want to use HIV itself, which carries obvious risks—yet, in animal trials, it's the one that has had the most success. But given the strength and volatility of HIV, this could be a very dangerous game.

## IMMUNE SYSTEM INVOLVEMENT

Although AIDS has had the unexpected "benefit" of bringing the immune system back into the forefront of medical science, we are now paying the price for having ignored it for so long. Although some diehard immunologists have been doing research on the immune system and its role on disease, it is only in recent years that there's been any appreciable amount of research into its various cellular functions. And what research there is tends to be very much in the pattern of the 1950s: how to find a drug, how to analyze the inner workings of the disease process, deconstruction—in other words, taking things apart and hoping to figure out how to put them back together, in one piece. What is not being taken into account is one of the most promising lines of treatment for AIDS, namely immunotherapy, or immune modulation. Various substances have been found that seem to work on components of the immune system, and it is in that line of research—as well in better understanding the underlying mechanisms—that the most hope lies for AIDS patients. To that end, it's necessary to study more patients who are able to control the progression of AIDS through their own immune strength and find what they have in common. Recent research suggests that stimulating natural killer cells might help the immune system fight HIV.

Immunotherapy has barely been touched in pharmaceutical companies' zeal to come up with a drug that will cure AIDS. But, given that AIDS involves a crippling of the immune system itself, it makes sense that nontoxic ways of shoring up immune-system functions could well hold the key to AIDS treatment. (See page 149 for a discussion of MGN-3 and AIDS.)

As we saw in Chapter 5, some scientists are experimenting with compounds that do shore up the immune system. It seems obvious that this research may take us closer to finding ways to control, if not cure, AIDS. Up to now, however, the research has been done mainly with cancer patients, partly because it is known that the immune system plays a role in cancer—though that role is not yet well understood. Gaining an understanding of how cancer—another disease whose incidence has increased dramatically in our modern world—works in the body will enable us to explore how immunotherapy can work to defeat the process.

# Chapter 10

# Cancer—
# A Civilized Killer

*"While there are several chronic diseases more destructive to life than cancer, none is more feared."*
—Charles H. Mayo (1865–1939), U.S. physician

Cancer. The very word is enough to conjure images of gaunt illness and failing strength; of being swept into painful therapies and brusque institutions. One in three people in North America will have cancer at some point in their lives, which means that nobody is exempt from its effects. Everyone knows someone—a parent, a friend, a colleague—who's been a victim. And every day, hundreds of people die. To get a visceral sense of it, imagine four fully loaded jumbo jets crashing each and every day, killing all passengers.

In spite of advances in virtually every area of medical science, cancer therapies have remained reactive and clumsy. We believe that within fifty years, many of the therapies now used to treat cancer—with the exception of surgery—will come to be regarded as we now regard the practice of bleeding that was commonly used 200 years ago. Occasionally more refined than they were before—particularly for systemic cancers like leukemia—they always come after the event, attacking the tumor, never affecting its development or acting on the disease process itself. The best "preventive" therapy that we've been able to come up with—in breast cancer, for instance—is to either administer high doses of a highly toxic and dangerous drug, tamoxifen, or offer high-risk women the "option" of having both breasts removed.

Can't we do better than this?

## A MODERN DISEASE?

Before the eighteenth century, cancer was rare. Ancient archeological remains indicate that tumors did not exist with any significant frequency. Anthropologists have examined Egyptian mummies, for example, in which some soft tissue is preserved, as well as skeletal remains of ancient cultures, and found no evidence of tumors in the bone. When cancer lodges in the bone, it creates a distinctive pattern—a pattern that is absent in old remains. A study of 100 mummies from Egypt, Alaska, and Peru did not turn up a single case of lung, breast, prostate, or bowel cancer[1]—all of which afflict modern populations with deadly regularity.

It's possible, of course, that those findings can be explained more by the virulence of other diseases that shortened human life spans than by the actual rarity of cancer. The average person rarely lived beyond the age of forty or fifty, and susceptibility to cancer increases with age. Furthermore, poor sanitation and unhygienic living conditions made other diseases, from cholera to typhus, both common and lethal. Infant and child mortality was high, and even the wealthy lived unhealthy lives—despite what Hollywood would have us believe. Lead was used in face powder and poisoned those who used it for too long, eventually creating ugly face lesions—or cancer. Smallpox and syphilis killed and maimed a huge number of people. On the other hand, smoking was rare, and the toxins and pollutants that are a daily part of our lives today were not a concern. Simple hygiene, adequate housing, and a decent diet were.

With modernity came cleanliness, good water, enhanced food

production and delivery, better homes, better health care and social services, and a generally improved quality of life—leading, in turn, to longer, healthier lives. With vaccination and antibiotics came a measure of freedom from disease, at least in the developed world. Diseases of prosperity, like heart disease and cancer, became the leading causes of death. Fifty years ago, the average life expectancy on this planet was forty-seven years. Now it's sixty-six, with people in developed countries living (on average) close to eighty years. The World Health Organization estimates that in the year 2025, the average life expectancy for the planet will be seventy-three. If there is a natural limit to the human life span, at this point we don't know what it is.[2] (Interestingly, your odds of living to a hundred increase the longer you live. Someone at eighty, for instance, has a greater chance of living another twenty years than does someone of sixty-five.) Overall, people live longer because they are healthier.

In spite of these rosy figures, the death toll from cancer—as well as heart disease and stroke—is steadily on the rise. Cancer respects neither youth, looks, talent, nor individual worth. It strikes seemingly at random, and nobody is immune to it. World-famous opera singers, politicians, brilliant thinkers, average people and children all get cancer. Some can afford more and better treatments, but, in the long run, it is the cancer and how quickly it spreads that determine how long a person will survive.

## RISING NUMBERS

Exact figures on the incidence of cancer in the United States are difficult to come by because the United States keeps no central data bank. What information there is has to be extrapolated from Bureau of Census figures and data collected through the National Cancer Institute's Surveillance Epidemiology and End Results (SEER), which follows only a few states.[3] Nonetheless, it is estimated that approximately 1.2 million new cases of cancer are diagnosed yearly in the United States, and the number is rising. Of these, over half a million die each year.

In 1980, new cancer cases were around 1 million yearly. By 1998, the figure had risen by a fifth. And Health Canada, the Canadian health agency that does keep tabs on this data (Canada and the United States are fairly similar in terms of disease patterns, or *epidemiology*), estimates that the incidence of cancer will rise another 30 percent over the next decade. Cancer risk increases with age, and Health Canada estimates that by the year 2010 half of all cancers diagnosed will be in the lung, prostate, colon, and rectum—in those aged seventy and older.[4] Under the age of forty, one's risk of cancer—all cancers—is one in fifty-eight for males and one in fifty-two for females. Between the ages of forty and sixty, that risk rises to one in thirteen and one in eleven, respectively. Above the age of sixty, the risk goes up to one in three (males) and one in four (females). Breast cancer is still a major risk for women, but lung cancer is rapidly becoming the number-one killer.

Beyond the numbers lies the human toll—in suffering, grieving families, broken lives, and death. Even though cardiovascular disease is officially the leading cause of death in the United States and Canada, it's cancer, the number-two killer, that's the grim reminder of mortality—and a reminder, too, of the shortcomings and failings of current medical practices. Although somewhat more refined than it used to be, cancer therapy, by and large, has not changed much in the last few decades. Tumors are removed surgically—which, in all fairness, is the only thing to do with them once they're in the body. Then, more often than not, the remaining cancer cells are attacked with brute force, with chemotherapy or radiation. Almost always, some cancer cells manage to survive and eventually propagate, usually with greater force. Cancer drugs are only slightly selective in terms of targets: they hit all fast-growing cells, including those in the hair, the skin, and the stomach lining. The "margin of safety is often very narrow," states one textbook.[5] Each cancer drug and treatment has a certain "kill rate." An 80-percent kill rate, for instance, gets rid of 80 percent of the cancer cells with each dose—and also of a lot of other cells that get in the way. It's been compared to forms of warfare where the harder the offensive, the greater the degree of collateral damage.

## THE CAUSES OF CANCER

Research has shown that approximately 25 percent—one out of four—of all cancers are "hard core." In other words, even the cleanest, healthiest living will not affect the incidence of these cancers because their basis is genetic. The remaining three-quarters, though, seem to be the result of a combination of environmental *carcinogens* (cancer-causing substances), genes, stress, and the person's ability to react to these factors. These figures may explain why we find so few instances of cancer in "tribal" populations and in the remains of ancient people. If only one out of four people got cancer—or perhaps fewer, in earlier times—the chances of actually finding that evidence would be slim. Future archeologists will have no difficulty in discovering cancer in our remains, however.

It's been estimated that about three-quarters of all cancers develop as a result of environmental chemicals. These include the ones that people expose themselves to voluntarily, like tobacco, alcohol, ultraviolet radiation, dyes, and cosmetics, as well more general ones such as pesticides, herbicides, solvents, plasticizers, asbestos, and aromatic hydrocarbons. Stress and the typical North American diet—which virtually ignores fruits, vegetables, and complex carbohydrates—are also implicated in the development of cancer.[6] Daily, new substances are discovered to be carcinogenic. In some cases, food additives and preservatives may be only a fraction of the cause, and in others, cancer might develop not because of the presence of any one of these substances alone but as a result of several of them reacting together in a vulnerable host. Modern life, replete with its many conveniences, has increased the risk of cancer dramatically. Although a few types of cancer, such as cervical and stomach cancer, have declined in developed countries, the more significant forms of the disease are on the rise. In fact, it is in developed countries, where the standard of living is higher, that cancer of the lung, breast, prostate, colon, and rectum have all become more frequent.[6]

## THE LIFE OF THE CELL

Cancer—whether it begins because of genetic factors, an excessive exposure to carcinogens, or a combination of both—doesn't happen overnight. But over time, for various reasons, the DNA in living cells becomes damaged. DNA at the best of times tends to be highly reactive and fragile.[6] Apparently, when DNA is damaged, it stimulates the production of cytokines—the same substances that signal "stop" to various processes set in place by the immune system, and that go awry in autoimmune disorders—and this may explain the diverse reactions, like inflammation and immune suppression, that certain carcinogenic substances can cause. The increase in cytokine production disrupts the normal cell "cycle."

Briefly, what happens in the normal cell cycle is this. At the beginning of the cycle, the cell slowly enlarges and makes a new protein. The DNA machinery turns on and begins to synthesize this new material. Finally, after getting bigger and bigger, the cell "decides" whether or not to divide. It's almost like walking into a dark room and deciding whether or not to press the light switch. You might decide not to turn on the light if there is a full moon and moonlight is streaming through the window. For the cell, it's not light but the presence of various proteins that influences its "decision" of whether to divide. When the cell does divide (called *mitosis*), it creates two exact duplicates of the original, with exactly the same chromosomes.

This cell cycle has various places where it can be disrupted. Exposure to toxic chemicals, certain illnesses—for example, chronic fatigue syndrome—and other factors can affect the cell cycle. At times, the cell can metaphorically "commit suicide," which in cells is an internally programmed process of cell death called *apoptosis*. Various external stimuli, such as high heat, bacterial toxins, chemotherapy, certain toxic chemicals, and ultraviolet light, can cause apoptosis.[6] Apoptosis somehow induces the cell membrane to change itself. There's evidence that it is the balance between cells dying naturally (apoptosis) or being killed (necrosis, or toxic cell death) and cells dividing (mitosis) that is affected by carcinogenic and toxic substances. Clearly, if more cells are dividing than dying, they start to proliferate and increase wildly—which is what they do when they create a tumor.

Cancer cells are fast, and they're primitive. "They multiply in a haphazard, unproductive way, fast and faster. They are called 'nondifferentiated' because they have no special function; cancer cells don't grow up to be skin cells or liver cells or nerve cells. They live only to reproduce again, take up more space," writes Sallie Tisdale, an acute-care nurse, in *The Sorcerer's Apprentice, Medical Miracles and Other Disasters.* "[They] are usually bigger than normal cells and they are shaped differently, amorphous. But they are also different from each other, each harking to a different call. No beehive here, no orderly rows or camps of cells all neatly tucked in together like logs in a loghouse. These queer birds go their own way, laughing, making ragged sheets and tangled nests. Most disturbing of all, they seem to thrive on trouble, growing in circumstances that would kill normal cells. In fact, abnormal conditions can speed the growth of cells and the bigger they get the hungrier they are."[5]

## FEEDING THE TUMOR

When a tumor forms, new blood vessels begin to form around it. This is called *neovascularization* or *angiogenesis.* The blood vessels feed the tumor by carrying in oxygen-rich blood to keep it going. Neovascularization can be prevented, or at least slowed, in most cases, by some combination of agents present in shark cartilage. That, in turn, prevents the tumor from growing. There's recently been much furor in newspapers and magazines (*Time's* cover story on May 18, 1998, for example), hailing the anti-angiogenic process as the new route to go in treating cancer. What's perhaps most extraordinary about this sudden "discovery" is how old it is and how long it's been around. I. William Lane—one of the authors of this book and a co-author of *Sharks Don't Get Cancer* and *Sharks Still Don't Get Cancer*—has spent the last two decades and more trying to interest the scientific and medical community in investigating this route. He has also personally spent enormous time and money researching it himself.[7,8] The cancer and arthritis patients he's helped have been grateful, even if the researchers have not. "Cancer cells are smart," this pioneer in shark cartilage likes to say. "They can get around chemotherapy. But they can't withstand starvation."

Shark cartilage appears to do exactly that: starve tumors of oxygen-rich blood through anti-angiogenesis. Some combination of the various components in shark cartilage prevents new blood vessels from forming. This, in turn, causes the tumor to starve and die. Why are new blood vessels the key to this process? "It is easier for tumor cells to penetrate newly developing capillaries than mature vessels," says *Sharks Don't Get Cancer.*[7] "Angiogenesis (the formation of new blood vessels) therefore provides a perfect route for tumor cells to move into the circulatory system, causing metastasis [spread of the cancer]. In addition, the tumor cells at the metastatic site must induce angiogenesis if they are to survive. This is more likely to occur when the primary tumor is highly angiogenic." This line of research is long overdue, given its solid scientific basis.

## IMMUNITY AND CANCER

The role of the immune system in cancer is not fully understood, though it undoubtedly plays a major role in preventing abnormal cellular activities on a regular basis throughout our lives. This idea, that the immune system prevents cancer many times within a person's lifetime, is known as the *immune surveillance hypothesis.* It proposes that cancer cells arise frequently but are rapidly "beaten down" by the immune system.[9] This concept—widely attributed to the late Lewis Thomas, who for many years headed the prestigious Sloan Kettering Cancer Institute in New York—was actually based on the work of Richmond Prehn and Joan Main, who discovered in 1957 that cancer cells could be detected by the body's own immune system.[10] Therefore, logically, it must be the vigilance—and actions—of the immune system that eliminates them.

For many years, however, fixed ideas about the immune system prevented the medical community from realizing that the immune system could be actively involved in getting rid of a tumor. For a long time, even the words used to describe tumor activity were passive, like saying the tumor "regressed," as though it magically just gave up and died. From AIDS patients, though, whose ravaged immune systems allow the development of opportunistic and rare cancers, we have learned that the immune system must indeed play a major and active part in keeping the millions of cells in our bodies "safe." According to the current theory, a cell-mediated immune response attacks anything it does not consider "self."

Where the theory falters is in describing how cancer cells—which are formed within a person's own body and would therefore be part of that person's "self" and carry the identifying "bar code," or MHC—could provoke an immune response. It has been shown, however, that many cancer cells carry unique non-MHC markers. These are the cancers that might be expected to provoke an immune response. It has also been shown that lymph nodes "downstream" from the cancer site usually contain some lymphocytes with the appropriate antibodies designed to "kill" those cells.[9] In that case, how does cancer slip by these cells? Cancer does happen, after all.

The simplest explanation is that the cancer grows so fast that the NK cells and cytotoxic (cell-killing) T cells are simply unable to keep up with them. Or possibly those cancer cells that have mutated, losing their MHC identity, can no longer be killed by the body's defensive cells. Another theory suggests that cancer cells might increase suppressor T cell response; yet another, that cancer cells might shed their antigens and "block" the receptors on the cytotoxic cells so they can't attack. The most logical explanation is that since most carcinogens are immune suppressants, NK cells become inactive and helpless in their wake.

There is some evidence that cancer cells themselves don't sit around and wait to be attacked. They may actually be quite active, giving out some sort of signal or substance that inhibits or interferes with NK cells and the immune response. If the immune system is working as it should be, NK and K cells should attack cancer cells and destroy them, quickly and efficiently. But as Dr. Mamdooh Ghoneum has demonstrated, all too often what happens is the reverse: the cancer cells kill *them*. Large and imposing, the cancer cell puts out an "arm" and encircles the NK cell and, essentially, eats it. This seems to happen particularly after chemotherapy or radiation, when the NK cells are weakened—which is an unfortunate result of these invasive cancer treatments. Furthermore, these processes themselves (chemotherapy and radiation) are strongly immunosuppressive—in much the same way that toxins, pollutants, and carcinogenic chemicals are immunosuppressive.[11] They *prevent* the body from being able to fend off viruses, or make antibodies in response to an external threat, by reducing the effectiveness of immune function.

For many years, it's been hoped that the immune system would aid in the battle against cancer. What chemotherapy and radiation left behind, the immune system would mop up. Many researchers, therefore, were flabbergasted to discover that chemotherapy actually *depresses* the immune system, rendering it useless in the face of bacterial attacks and viral onslaughts. "To this day too little attention is paid to this unfortunate linkage (that of ostensibly therapeutic agents used to combat cancer, namely chemotherapy, causing suppression of the immune system)," writes one immunologist, "leaving an indeterminate number of chemotherapy patients unnecessarily immune depressed, at risk for opportunistic infections, and, possibly, cancer recurrences."[11]

## USING THE IMMUNE SYSTEM TO CURE CANCER

Given the sheer number of cells in our body and the millions of interactions they engage in, as well as the increasing numbers of stresses, both personal and environmental, that the whole system is exposed to, it is surprising in many ways that cancers don't develop more often than they do. Obviously, the immune system does play a part: as one ages and one's immune system becomes less active, cancers develop more. Studies on mice have demonstrated that as the animal ages, the ability of its leukocytes to kill tumors becomes less efficient, and cancer cells are killed too slowly. The reverse is true for "young leukocytes," which have a high degree of anti-tumor activity.[12] That may explain why traditional methods of eradicating cancer are reasonably successful in children. Perhaps children's immune systems and leukocytes are more effective than those of older patients at "catching" the cancerous cells left behind after treatment.

Immunotherapy has not received the attention it should have in the past few decades. Too often, the prevailing "fashion" in medicine has been intent on eradicating the source of disease—the way antibiotics created the idea that once the offending bacteria were destroyed, the person would no longer be sick. Unfortunately, cancer statistics show that this approach has been of marginal benefit at best. Public relations departments of cancer agencies all over the world paint glowing reports of successes and improvements in treatment, point to people who've lived five, ten, twenty years after having had cancer, and put a positive spin on the grim statistics. But the statistics ignore the reality that the basis for any success we've had lies largely in better diagnostic and screening techniques—detecting tumors earlier, while they are smaller. The actual therapeutic approach to cancer has not changed in many decades. Fierce territorialism on the part of much of the cancer "establishment" has maintained the status quo, as have peer pressure and genuine fears of legal ramifications for individual physicians who go outside accepted strict treatment protocols. Credit must be given to the many individual clinicians who, on a daily basis, try to do their best for their patients, however much in the minority they might appear to be.

Patients themselves have been the driving force behind many of the advances and changes that have been made. And thanks largely to the press—which has kept people informed of discoveries such as shark cartilage—as well as other information sources like the Internet, ordinary people have been able to increase their choices and become involved in their own treatment. Information, as they say, is political, and for too many years experts have "hoarded" information and kept the language of science inaccessible to anyone other than other experts.

For a few years there was much excitement about using interferon, one of the cytokines in the immune system's arsenal against viruses, as an agent to stimulate or modulate the immune system. These agents—which, it was hoped, would be true biological response modifiers, or BRMs—have been a giant failure as anticancer agents. Even though biotechnological techniques synthesized the substance so that it was nearly 99-percent pure, it was still not pure *enough* and caused severe side effects in those who took it: kidney failure, capillary leaking syndrome, vomiting, and nausea, among others.[13] Nevertheless, it is a promising line of therapy that has barely been examined.

Therapeutically, what this means is that cancer patients desperately seeking cures and treatments should not automatically fall for anything that calls itself an immune booster. There is more going on with cancer than an immune system lag or slowdown. Of course, given that the incidence of cancer does increase with age, a lackluster performance on the part of the immune system does play a part, but it's important to realize which part(s) and what mechanisms are at work. We tend to like simple generalizations: a strong immune system is "good," a weak one is "bad"—and to some extent this is true. But immune "dampening" techniques with steroid drugs used to treat autoimmune disorders have been shown to offer merely symptom relief. They do nothing to address the cause. A fibrosis type of illness like scleroderma, for instance, is probably caused by cytokines and fibroblasts, not by the whole immune system. By the same token, attempting to "kickstart" the entire immune system in order to treat cancer—especially with unproven and possibly quack cures that have more public relations behind them than science—may well end up being counterproductive and possibly even dangerous. To fight tumors with immunity, it's necessary to engage NK and other specific cells.

The balancing act that is immunity has built-in checks and balances. It has different components, different parts, each with separate roles and responsibilities. It's important to work *with* the immune system intelligently. If we want to enhance its tumor-destroying capacities, we need to give it the right ammunition and the right equipment. Otherwise, it's like the cartoon showing a group of housepainters being given computers. Having no idea what to do with them, they proceed to use them as stepladders so they can reach the high parts.

Scientists have known for twenty years that the specific immune-system cells that particularly react to tumors are called NK—natural killer—cells. Knowing the "troops" would seem to be a good starting point for issuing the right equipment. But the cancer establishment has continued to rely on traditional treatments, including radiation and chemotherapy, that actually depress the strength and activity of NK cells. In the next chapter, we will look at some research that could turn cancer therapy on its ear.

# Part Four

---

# Cooperating
# With the
# Immune System

# Chapter 11

# Natural Killer Cells, MGN-3, Cancer, and AIDS

*"In treating a patient, let your first thought be to strengthen his natural vitality."*

—Rhazes (850–923), Persian physician

Look at the sky at night and think about the millions of stars, planets, quasars, galaxies, comets, and other bodies in the universe. Even with a telescope, it's impossible to get any real sense of its immensity and complexity. Similarly, the immune system, with its myriad connections, cross-links, and responses, is so incredibly complicated that it is impossible to generalize about it. Over the past few decades, science has given us a much clearer picture of how the various components of immunity work—largely because of AIDS, which has been a grim reminder of just how important the immune system is. It has become increasingly obvious to what extent we would fall prey to opportunistic infections, rare cancers, and bacteria without the vigilance of our immune system. We now know that the various lymphocytes and phagocytes in our lymph nodes, spleen, and bone marrow play a role that is essential to health.

To review briefly, all living creatures—from the lowly sponge all the way to humans—have various ways of reacting to a physiological threat, whether it's a bacterium like typhoid, a parasite such as the one that causes malaria, or a virus like smallpox and HIV. The body's first line of defense always tends to be generalized and nonspecific: inflammation, macrophages that "eat" invading bacteria, and so on. Over time, if this line of defense proves inadequate, the immune system sends in its "big guns." Depending on the source of the problem, the heavy artillery might involve humoral immunity—mostly B cells, attacking invaders in the blood—or cellular immunity—mostly T cells, attacking the cell directly. In cancer, however, the real defense is comprised of the natural killer (NK) cells and cytotoxic T lymphocytes (CTLs) first discussed in Chapter 3. NK cells and CTL cells have a remarkable relationship with cancer, one that needs to be understood if new and perhaps more effective directions in cancer therapy are going to be followed.

## CELLULAR CANCER KILLERS

NK cells, as we saw in Chapter 3, are a cranky, short-tempered bunch. They don't like viruses and hate tumors, the mere sight of which makes them go on the offensive. NK cells were first noticed in the mid-1970s when immunologists realized that there seemed to be an immune-system defense against cancer that behaved differently from T and B cells.[1] Repeated studies have shown that people with cancer who have high rates of NK-cell activity also have high rates of survival.[2] For instance, Spanish researchers who were studying surgical results found that in forty patients who had had curative surgery for colorectal tumors, NK-cell activity was in direct proportion to the progression of their illness.[3] In other words, the more NK-cell activity there was, the better the outcome for the patient. Similarly, a study at the University of Pittsburgh that followed ninety women in Stage I or Stage II breast cancer found that "NK cell activity was a strong predictor of disease outcome" when "outcome" was defined in its most basic form as recurrence of cancer.[4] These are only a few of the many studies that have found NK-cell activity to be directly correlated with cancer-cell destruction, and, by extension, longer life for cancer patients.

This NK-cell anticancer activity is referred as "natural cytotoxicity." In other words, NK cells produce a natural toxin, emanating from the immune system, that can attack cancer cells on a cellular level. But as we have already seen, powerful chemicals are directly involved in immunosuppression—whether they're in cigarette smoke, industrial waste, or chemotherapy drugs. In fact, many standard cancer therapies are a double-edged sword. On the one hand, they might get rid of most of the cancer cells, but on the other hand, they are preventing the immune system from doing its job. If virtually all the current standard treatments for cancer reduce NK activity, and reduced NK activity reduces the body's ability to fight cancer, doesn't it make sense to try to *increase* the potency of NK cells and thereby use them in therapy? As the authors of a literature review on the subject of NK cells and cancer write: "NK . . . cells, through the use of immune biologic modifiers, have been demonstrated to have a therapeutic role in the treatment of human cancers."[5]

## TREATMENTS LAG BEHIND RESEARCH

Ideally, the knowledge about NK cells' anticancer activity should be put to use in the treatment of cancer, and the workings of the immune system itself should be taken into account when chemotherapy and radiation treatment are considered. As the authors quoted above conclude: "Further studies are required to determine the optimal dosages and combinations of chemotherapeutic agents, the timing of surgery, and the adjuvant use of immune biologic response modifiers."[5] They conclude that "an increasing awareness and understanding" in this area could contribute to promising anticancer therapies for the future.

As anyone who's ever had direct experience of the cancer "establishment" knows, however, these promising avenues of therapy have played only a minimal part in the treatment of cancer.

However promising they may be, they've been ignored—pushed to the back of the experimental funding wagon. Regardless of how many studies have indicated the probable effectiveness of these strategies, regardless of how many researchers have urged that these avenues should be explored, standard cancer therapies have remained, in essence, static for a very long time. Every once in a while some development in gene therapy or an exciting research idea makes its way to the front pages (as interferon and inter-leukin-2 did), but almost as quickly, it disappears from public notice. Small biotechnology firms have made some promising advances, but nearly all are in the early detection and diagnosis of cancerous tissue, not in therapy. This is not "winning" the war against cancer; it's stalemate.

Of course it is true that many recent developments in cancer research have increased the odds of surviving cancer longer. And some early screening—a good example is the Pap test for detecting cervical cancer—has translated into enormous successes. But in spite of the advances, oncology—cancer medicine—remains one of the most laboratory-driven and technology-based specialties around. In the treatment of just about any other medical problem, there is at least *some* recognition that the person—not just the tumor or the laboratory findings—is of some importance. How the person *feels*, his or her stress levels, social network, dietary habits, level of activity, and general level of health, as well as immune, res-piratory, and digestive system function, are acknowledged as play-ing a role. Most family doctors and practitioners of many other medical specialties do talk to patients about lifestyle choices—about exercise and smoking, for instance—and about becoming active participants in their own recovery. But somehow, with can-cer, the medical process and the use of treatment protocols have subverted the whole idea of medicine and turned the process of dealing with this terrible, frightening illness into a purely biologi-cal endeavor.

Individual doctors might occasionally counsel their patients about diet, stress, or exercise; however, as a whole, the cancer establishment has been woefully negligent in terms of allowing patients to feel that they are participating in their treatment—and in terms of treating patients well. Dr. Bernie Siegal, himself a medical doctor and author of the popular *Love, Medicine & Miracles*, writes: "As doctors, many of us have cultivated our detachment so effectively that our patients find us completely inhuman. The truth without compassion is hostility. I had a patient come to my office the other day who had had a mammogram in Spain, and she told me that when the time came for her to get the results, both the technician and the physician walked out and embraced her before telling her the news that she would need surgery. When she came to his country for treatment, she was shocked by the difference in physicians. The first surgeon she was referred to talked to her with his back toward her as he completed a chart, and got angry at her for asking how her breast would look after surgery. She found a similar coldness in the radiology suite she visited."[6]

Some of this detachment—outright cruelty, according to some patients—might be due to the extent to which cancer therapy is laboratory-driven. From the diagnostic tests to the biopsy results, what doctors do is dictated by "treatment protocols"—guidelines for each and every type of tumor, instructions on what the standard forms of treatment should be. Use this-and-that kind of chemo or radiation or surgery, in such-and-such a way. Individual physicians' hands are tied—and they are further confined by their fear of legal consequences should they deviate from the "norm."

There's evidence that *chronotherapy*—the timing of interventions and therapies—is important in treatment. Has this entered into actual practice? No. For women, there's evidence that scheduling certain treatments for breast cancer at specific points in the woman's monthly menstrual cycle makes the therapy more effective. Is this taken into account? Of course not. There's even evidence that some drugs work better for some people when given at certain times of day. But these ideas have not penetrated, even marginally, into clinical practice. There is solid evidence that diet, exercise, laughter, and other lifestyle issues play a part in healing, yet only a few doctors and nurses discuss these issues with their cancer patients. Patient issues have largely gotten lost in the gears of the giant cancer "machine."

Cancer treatment remains focused on the cancer itself—on eradicating it. Small wonder, then, that so many patients have taken matters into their own hands—flocked to complementary therapists and undertaken their own treatment protocols in addition to whatever's been recommended to them by the cancer medical establishment. Terrified patients are, more often than not, pushed into ill-understood procedures that are described in cold medical terminology and risk/benefit ratios. Sick and unable to make clear decisions, they're treated in high-tech environments with procedures that are rarely explained adequately.

## MGN-3, A BIOLOGICAL RESPONSE MODIFIER

Back in Chapter 5, we introduced Dr. Mamdooh Ghoneum's research on Arabinoxylan Compound, or MGN-3. Dr. Ghoneum found that MGN-3 influences NK cells to double or triple their activity, resulting in the death of many more cancer cells. The fact that it affects the NK cells' activity rather than their numbers makes it a true biological response modifier, or BRM—a nontoxic substance that has measurable effects on biological responses, such as those of the immune system.

### The MGN-3 Mechanism

Under the microscope, NK cells are nearly indistinguishable from T and B cells. But unlike the other two, NK cells contain tiny black granules that are their "bullets." Without these granules, they have little killing power; they're like a gun that's been emptied of ammunition. About 10 percent of the NK cell is made up of cytoplasm containing these granules.

"Cancer patients have as many NK cells as anybody else," says Dr. Ghoneum. "But their NK cells don't have granules. Cancer cells may degranulate NK cells." What MGN-3 does is put the granules back into existing cells: *regranulate* NK cells. Remember, the compound doesn't increase the *number* of cells but the potency of the ones that are there—as though weak and sickly NK cells had begun lifting weights and become strong and able again.

Exactly how the NK cells bind to the cancer cell is still a bit of a mystery. What is known is that the NK cell-tumor interaction proceeds through several stages. "First," says Dr. Ghoneum, "there is an effector-to-target recognition." A cellular "alarm" goes off: Emergency! This triggers the activation of the NK cells, which race over to see what the problem is. Finally, each NK cell releases the granules that, like bullets, punch holes in the cancer cells—"shoots" them dead. (See Figure 11.1 on page 142.) "You easily see the holes in the body of the cancer cell," Dr. Ghoneum says. "In less than five minutes, when the NK cell is working at top speed, the cancer cell is dead." And with MGN-3, any NK cells that are unable to do anything about proliferating cancer cells become rejuvenated, strengthened—and go back to work killing cancer cells with renewed vigor. (See Figure 11.2 on page 143.)

The extraordinary thing about MGN-3, however, is not its ability to increase the fighting strength of NK cells *in vitro* or in the aging rats residing in Dr. Ghoneum's laboratory, but in its power to fight cancer in living human beings. In real live *sick* human beings.

As we've seen, the true cancer-fighting powerhouses of the immune system are the NK and CTL cells. Other cells, such as B cells, may kill cancer—but that's because in an emergency situation like cancer, all the troops come out to help. If there's a major disaster in your town, you don't say, "I'm not a relief worker so I can't do anything"; everybody pitches in and does what they can, even if it's only dialing 911. In the immune system, the only cells that are specifically designed to kill tumor cells are the NK and CTL cells; the others simply pitch in when things get really touch-and-go.

Like well-trained commandos toting automatic weapons, NK cells blast away at tumor cells with the granules inside their cytoplasm. The problem is that the cancer itself—as well as stressful treatments like chemo, radiation, and surgery, and the stress of

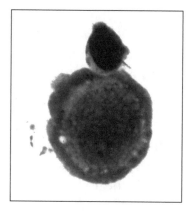

**A.** The NK cell (top) attaches itself to the cancer cell (bottom).

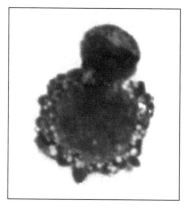

**B.** The NK cell injects a bullet-like granule into the cancer cell.

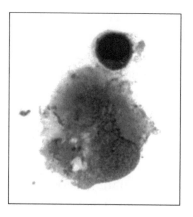

**C.** With the cancer cell dead, the NK cell disengages itself and goes back on the prowl.

**Figure 11.1.** A natural killer (NK) cell killing a cancer cell.

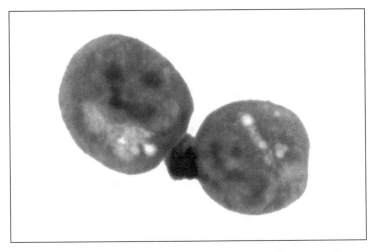

**A.** The NK cell attaches itself to two cancer cells at one time.

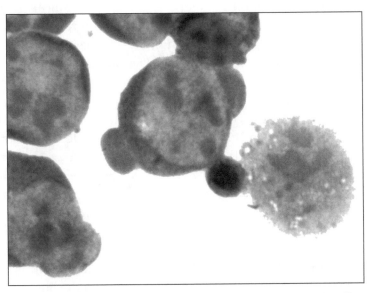

**B.** After killing one cancer cell, the NK cell disengages itself and moves on to attack the second cancer cell.

**Figure 11.2.** An aggressive natural killer (NK) cell killing cancer cells.

being ill in the first place—all *suppress* the immune system. So the shock troops of immunity suddenly find themselves stripped of their ammunition, degranulated—left helpless at a time when they're most needed. As the immune system reels under the assaults it undergoes with cancer, the "bullets" in the commandos' guns—the granules in the NK cells—aren't there. These feisty killers find themselves not only unarmed but vulnerable to attack from large, menacing cancer cells. "Many people don't know that when the immune system is low, the NK cells or macrophages, cytotoxic lymphocytes that are supposed to kill the cancer cell, can't. The cancer cell kills them," says Dr. Ghoneum.

## MGN-3 and Interferon

The idea of using an immune modulator, or biological response modifier, as an immunotherapeutic agent to treat cancer is not a new one. Years ago, when it was found that interferon—one of the cytokines naturally produced by the immune system—is able to stimulate the immune system to work more effectively against cancer and viruses, there was much excitement. The excitement just as quickly died down when it was discovered that the substance could not be artificially produced in pure enough form to be useful—its side effects were unacceptable. A decade later another cytokine, interleukin-2 (IL-2), created the same buzz. "Another champion," says Dr. Ghoneum. "Another cytokine, same family, and many doctors gave it to their patients. Again, confronted with the same problem of enormous side effects." Interleukin, to be effective, has to be given in very high doses and causes unpleasant side effects, such as nausea and vomiting, as well as more serious ones like kidney failure. In addition, making interleukin is very expensive, and treating even one patient with it in the hospital can cost as much as $100,000.[7]

IL-2 can be tolerated—but only in such small doses that its presence is ineffective. Dr. Ghoneum has found, however, that adding MGN-3 to low doses of IL-2 has a dramatic and synergistic impact. (*Synergistic* means that two substances used together are more effective than the sum of their individual effects.) MGN-3, a simple, nontoxic compound made from processed rice bran, is not only well tolerated on its own but makes a powerhouse out of low doses of interferon. Simultaneously, it regranulates NK cells and gives them back their "firepower." MGN-3, which has been used in Japan for about a decade by tens of thousands of Japanese cancer patients, seems to enhance the power of the body's own cytokines, which for years has been suspected to play a part in the regression of cancerous tumors.

In research with cancer patients, MGN-3 has been shown to be safe and to have virtually no side effects. Its impact on cancer cells, however, is remarkable—both speedy and measurable. And unlike most so-called immune-boosting agents, whose hype declares them equally effective against everything from hives to herpes, MGN-3 has been quietly and scientifically tested, *in vitro*, in the laboratory and with human subjects, for years in the United States. (As discussed in the Preface, it was one of Dr. Ghoneum's patients who brought MGN-3 to the authors' attention in the first place.) The effects of MGN-3 and the results of studies done with it aren't in the public-relations domain but are found in peer-reviewed journals and in abstracts from medical conferences, like the Annual Meeting of the American Association for Cancer Research and the International Conference on AIDS. Perhaps most important, this is not a product that professes to have a general enhancing effect on immunity—which, as we have seen, can have detrimental effects: autoimmune diseases are the result of an *overactive* immune system. Rather, MGN-3 works in a specific way. It increases the activity, not the numbers, of NK cells—the body's first line of defense against cancer.

## RESEARCH ON MGN-3 AND CANCER PATIENTS

Clinical trials have demonstrated the efficacy of MGN-3 with simple statistical power. Next, you will learn the results of studies that examined the effect of this substance on cancer.

## A Study of Different Cancers

Eleven randomly selected cancer patients, all undergoing the standard therapies for their particular kind of cancer, were also given three grams of MGN-3 orally each day.[7] Three of the patients had prostate cancer; three, ovarian; three, breast; and two, multiple myeloma. Their treatments had ranged from Lupron (for prostate cancer) to surgery, radiation, chemotherapy, and bone marrow transplant (for one multiple myeloma patient). Dr. Ghoneum and his team drew blood from each patient before treatment, then again at two weeks post-treatment, and thereafter at monthly intervals. NK activity and tumor-associated antigens specific to each type of cancer were measured. With respect to the tumor-associated antigens—the biological markers used to determine the amount of cancer in the patient's system—these were the results:

• Prostate-specific antigen, or PSA, was used as the marker for prostate cancer. All patients had a significant decline in their levels of PSA. Two patients showed a very rapid decline and achieved normal PSA after a few months of treatment with MGN-3. These patients' PSA levels started out at 7.9 and 6.8, and went down to below 0.2 and 0.1, respectively.

• Two of the three patients with ovarian cancer showed a significant decline in CA 125, the marker for ovarian cancer. The initial decrease was rapid (one month) and levels of CA 125 reached normal (35 units) three to four months post-treatment.

• The two patients with multiple myeloma (a rare and lethal form of cancer that affects the bone marrow) had very different tumor-associated antigens; however, both showed reductions with MGN-3

• The three patients with breast cancer started out with low CA 15-3 levels (the marker for breast cancer) and this did not change with MGN-3. However, their computerized tomography (CT) scans were negative.

NK-cell activity in these patients was also measured. Overall, patients showed a low level of basal NK activity at the outset, which in two weeks increased almost threefold. Nine of the eleven patients had a significant increase in their NK activity after treatment with MGN-3. In their discussion, Dr. Ghoneum and his colleagues write that "[these] data demonstrate that [MGN-3] is a promising anti-cancer agent as manifested by a significant decline of TAA (tumor-associated antigen) in eight out of eleven patients with different types of malignancies." Some cancers, like prostate and ovarian, responded quickly; multiple myeloma took longer.

**Breast Cancer**

Five patients with breast cancer were each given three grams of MGN-3 daily. The results, presented at an American Association for Cancer Research Special Conference in 1995, are outlined below.

• Patients started out with very low levels of basal NK-cell activity (13.5 percent to 34.9 percent) at effector-to-target (NK cell to cancer cell) ratios of 12:1 and 100:1. The NK-cell activity was significantly enhanced by MGN-3 treatment at the same effector-to-target ratios.

• Increases in NK-cell activity were noted as early as one to two weeks post-treatment.

• NK-cell activity further increased over time. Most important, this increase was maintained over a period of years, in contrast with the temporary increase that has occurred with many other immune stimulants.

• Four patients who participated early in the study are in complete remission.

**Various Cancers**

A study of twenty-seven cancer patients was presented at the 87th Annual Meeting of the American Association for Cancer

Research in Washington DC in April 1996. Seven of the patients had breast cancer; seven, prostate; eight, multiple myeloma; three, leukemia; and two, cervical cancer. The study showed that patients began with low levels of NK-cell activity (10.8 percent to 40 percent). NK-cell activity steadily increased after two weeks of daily treatment with three grams of MGN-3. All patients showed an increase in their NK-cell activity. In the patients with breast, prostate, and cervical cancers and leukemia, NK-cell activity more than doubled; in those with multiple myeloma they quintupled (became five times as active), going from 100 percent to 537 percent.

NK-cell activity continued to rise in the months after treatment (it was measured at three and six months). Dr. Ghoneum concludes, undramatically, in his abstract's concluding remarks that "the high augmentory [enhancing] effect of MGN-3 makes it a promising immunotherapeutic agent for treating cancer."

## Case Studies

The previous discussions provided strong statistical evidence of the power of MGN-3. The following case histories show how this substance helped two individuals with cancer.

### Multiple Myeloma

The first case study is that of a fifty-eight-year-old man, a physician with no previous history of cancer, who developed multiple myeloma in October 1990. Multiple myeloma, also called myelomatosis, is a rare and often lethal form of cancer characterized by uncontrollable growth of cancer cells and a disorder in the function of B cells in the bone marrow. He had severe pain in his lower back (the disease causes bone tissue to be destroyed) and his blood tests showed clear abnormalities. The patient was started on physical therapy for the pain in his back, and on chemotherapy. He became increasingly ill and bedridden, at which time he was started on interferon alfa-2a, which has been occasionally successful in treating multiple myeloma. After some initial improvement, the cancer did not regress significantly.

In March 1992, the patient stopped all other medications and was started on MGN-3.[8] No other drugs were given at this point, since the chemotherapy no longer appeared to be working. The oncologists couldn't do anything more for him, in other words. The patient was then given three grams of MGN-3 a day. Within twenty-four hours, his marker levels dropped and "subsequently [went] from 150 mg/day, to 30, 20, 10 and reached undetectable levels at seventeen months post-treatment," writes Dr. Ghoneum.

Immunoglobulins (produced by B cells, as you'll recall from Chapter 3) were also monitored. "There was a sustained gradual elevation of all three immunoglobulins (IgG, IgA, and IgM)," and the patient regained normal ability to produce immunoglobulins. NK-cell activity was measured a month later, after the patient had stopped taking all drugs. Results showed an increase in NK-cell activity, which was maintained six months post-treatment. This increase in activity was noticed at all effector-to-target cell ratios. In other words, the ratios of NK ("effector") cells to cancer ("target") cells, indicating that the NK cells were destroying the cancer cells, were 12:1, 25:1, 50:1, and 100:1—which would seem to indicate pretty strongly that NK cells play a major role in the destruction of leukemic cancer cells.

### Ovarian Cancer

The second case report is of a fifty-three-year-old woman with ovarian cancer—the same cancer that killed actress Gilda Radner. Previously healthy, the woman was admitted to the hospital with swollen breasts and a distended stomach. Ovarian cancer was diagnosed in both ovaries in February 1993. Following surgery to remove her ovaries, she went through a course of chemotherapy and, additionally, was given three grams of MGN-3 per day.[9] The average patient with this type of cancer takes up to four months to normalize after chemotherapy; in this lady's case, she went into complete remission after two. "[A] combination of chemotherapy with concurrent use of MGN-3 resulted in shortening of the peri-od to achieve complete clinical remission," writes Dr. Ghoneum in his conclusion. The patient evidently agreed. After stopping chemo, she continued with MGN-3.

Chemotherapeutic drugs, as we know, are immunosuppres-sants. Whether they reduce the number of immune cells or simply make them less active is not yet clear, but what is obvious is that adding a biological response modifier, such as MGN-3, can keep the immune reaction more "normal" and enable the body's own defenses to fight the cancer as well. NK-cell activity in this patient returned to normal after only three weeks of therapy with MGN-3. Since MGN-3 has no discernible side effects, is not toxic, and does not affect liver enzymes, adding it to standard cancer treat-ments would seem to be a fairly benign—and logical—route to go.

## INCLUDING THE IMMUNE SYSTEM IN CANCER TREATMENT

"The immune system needs to be taken seriously," says Dr. Ghoneum flatly. Even under optimal conditions, when we're not sick, the world we live in works as a kind of immunosuppressive agent. Air pollution, chemical carcinogens, toxins used to treat our crops . . . the cumulative effects of these on the immune system are immense. Then there are all the things people do to themselves, from smoking cigarettes to exposing themselves to the ultraviolet rays of the sun. The average North American diet, too, is not known for its health-giving properties. And we've all felt the effects of stress on our lives.

But cancer patients, in addition to the multiple stresses of illness and the physical strain of the treatments they have to undergo, have an added barrier to immune health: the treatments themselves, espe-cially radiation and chemotherapy, depress the immune system even further. (Remember that some researchers, in order to test immune-suppressed laboratory mice, subject them to radiation.) Under these circumstances, it seems like sheer folly not to at least try to help the immune system with a biological response modifier such as MGN-3, which has been shown to be effective in enhancing the activity of NK cells.

If cancer is very far advanced, using MGN-3 alone may not be enough. After all, it's taken as long as twenty years for the malignancy to develop. Years of slightly maladaptive or inappropriate responses and long periods of abnormal immune-system activity are what led to the cancer in the first place. Waiting too long can be fatal. Surgery, if the cancer is a solid tumor, is usually the safest bet; the tumor has to be removed. With systemic cancers, chemotherapy or other processes that kill the cancer cells may be called for. But in the early stages, it's difficult to say with any certainty what the exact route should be. Each person will be different—not only in terms of risk tolerance but in the progression of the disease.

If you decide to use MGN-3, the dose now being used by people with cancer is three grams a day for two to four weeks, and then one gram a day as a maintenance dose. It may even be possible to use MGN-3 as a preventive—for people who work in toxic environments like factories or dry-cleaning establishments, for instance—though this has not been established yet. Ideally, you should consult with a health-care professional whom you trust—someone who understands how disease works and, most important, who understands that the entire person is involved in the disease and that using the power of the immune system to regain health is vital.

## MGN-3 AND AIDS

An unexpected bonus of MGN-3 research has been its potential for treating AIDS. Dr. Ghoneum has found that *in vitro* MGN-3 effectively prevents HIV-1 replication. Blood was drawn from three healthy individuals, and certain blood cells were then "infected" with HIV.[10] Half the sample was treated with MGN-3, while the other was left as a control. At the end of the incubation period, it was found that MGN-3 inhibited the replication of HIV-1 in a dose-dependent manner—in other words, at low concentrations the effect was small, but at higher concentrations the production of

HIV-1 antigen was reduced by as much as 75 percent. This means that the immune system successfully fought off HIV, with the assistance of MGN-3.

Subsequently, blood from five AIDS patients was treated in the same way and the number of syncytia (a mass of cells like a tumor) measured. MGN-3 "significantly inhibited syncytia formation," writes Dr. Ghoneum. He presented his results at the XIth International Conference on AIDS in Vancouver, Canada, in July 1996.

"Side effects are one of the biggest problems in using anti-HIV agents," says Dr. Ghoneum. "The prolonged use of various drugs, like AZT, is associated with severe toxicity." As with antibiotics, resistance develops to anti-HIV drugs, which is why medical experts now suggest using multiple-drug therapies against AIDS. MGN-3, being a biological response modifier, acts on the immune system rather than attacking the virus, and thus the virus cannot develop resistance to it. Given the tenacity with which HIV has resisted all our efforts to control and treat it, if MGN-3 can indeed halt its progression as these results indicate it might, then we are on the brink of a major clinical breakthrough with extraordinary social, medical, and public health consequences.

Remember, you heard it here first.

# Chapter 12

# Enhancing Your Immune Power

*"Physicians are inclined to engage in hasty generalizations.*
*Possessing a natural or acquired distinction, endowed with*
*a quick intelligence, an elegant and facile conversation . . .*
*the more eminent they are . . . the less leisure they have for*
*investigative work . . . Eager for knowledge . . . they are apt to*
*accept too readily attractive but inadequately proven theories."*

—Louis Pasteur (1822–1895), French scientist

We've known for years that the immune system plays a role in maintaining health and that its efficient functioning keeps us free of virulent diseases, from viruses to cancer. We still don't know the exact details of how that is accomplished. This is because research into the immune system was out of favor for many years and gained ground only with the advent of AIDS. AIDS made it obvious that the immune system's healthy functioning was essential to health, since this virus that could ravage the immune system would also kill anyone who contracted it. But even the burst of research that resulted from AIDS couldn't make up for years of neglect, and much of our knowledge about the immune system is still both oversimplified and incomplete.

Today, we're starting to realize that the immune system is like a finely tuned and complicated instrument that needs a delicate touch. Mark Lappé, a nationally recognized immunologist, writes in the *Tao of Immunology*, "[Various] findings underscore the tightrope we walk in maintaining an adaptive level of immunological fitness."[1] He suggests that this complex balance needs to be seen in a more Eastern sense than Western medicine has hitherto done: as a state of dynamic equilibrium. The prevailing view, in contrast, is that the immune system is some kind of mechanical device that needs adjustment. Unfortunately, health care is a giant industry that is about as amenable to changing direction as a charging rhino. Once something becomes accepted practice, altering it is very difficult.

Take ulcers. For years, doctors prescribed antacids, bland diets, even surgery to treat gastric ulcers. The therapy wasn't terribly successful, but it was accepted protocol. The news that most ulcers were due to a bacterium was initially greeted with skepticism and then completely ignored. (No doubt the drug companies that manufactured acid-reducing drugs had a hand in this.) It took nearly twenty years, but finally the evidence was so overwhelming it had to be accepted. It's the same with most medical practices. Once something gets into the medical textbooks and into clinical practice, it requires an enormous amount of time and scientific proof to bring about change in the therapeutic process. (Ironically, *therapeutics*, which means the art and science of treating disease, comes from a Greek word meaning "inclined to serve." Exactly who is being served is questionable; it's certainly not the patient much of the time.)

The immune system—this vast network of cells that maintains the integrity of the self—is, we now know, essential to good health and life itself. As we have seen, there is no such thing as total immunity. We cannot be totally protected against external threats—whether they are disease-causing microorganisms, environmental contaminants, or stress. It is possible, however, for each one of us to increase our immune power.

## EXERCISE AND DIET

There are few lifestyles as unhealthy as that of the average stressed, overworked American family. Racing from work to pick up children at school or daycare, eating junk food, flopping exhausted in front of the television set at the end of the day—few strategies could be as detrimental to health and the immune system as this. However, if you work out regularly, you can prevent or curtail ailments from colds to cancer, says health and science professor David Nieman in *The Exercise-Health Connection*.[2] Regular, moderate exercise, which doesn't have to be difficult—a brisk half-hour walk every day will do—has been shown to affect the immune system and to reduce stress. The key is moderate and regular.

Extreme exercise actually has harmful effects on the immune system. Researchers at the Copenhagen Muscle Research Centre have found that heavy training, such as that engaged in by professional athletes, reduces the levels of T cells and NK cells for as long as twenty hours after the session.[3] Since professional athletes rarely stop their training for that long, this could have serious long-term health consequences. Chronic training, in fact, appears to lead to a kind of chronic condition all its own, similar to chronic fatigue syndrome.

Very few of us, however, are in any danger of that syndrome, since most of us tend to exercise too little, not too much. This is a big mistake. There is solid evidence that the low-level stress caused by an exercise program actually stimulates antibody protection and maintains our levels of NK activity. It appears to be our ability to cope with stress that is at stake when it comes to immune health, and, like muscles that grow stronger with sustained low-level exercise, the immune-system cells similarly become more "muscled" and fit.

Diet also has a strong impact on how well our body functions in general. In particular, antioxidants, such as vitamins C and E, have recently been shown to have life-enhancing and health-giving properties. All living cells, like people, need food to survive. For cells, nutrition equals oxygen, without which they die in very short order. Oxygen is constantly involved in chemical cellular reactions that then, in turn, create other, unstable molecules.[4] These free radicals, as they're called (think of them as wandering, aimless people who have nothing better to do than get into trouble), can cause damage unless they are "caught up" by antioxidants (think of these as social workers).

Where do we get antioxidants? In vitamins C and E and carotenoids such as beta-carotene. Taking megadoses of supplements is not really a solution because they can cause problems for some people. It's better to eat lots of fruits and vegetables, a minimum of five servings a day—and supplement as necessary. This dietary practice has positive effects on everything from heart disease to weight control. An added bonus of getting all those extra vitamins and fiber is the "boost" these give us in fighting stress and in fighting off the effects of environmental toxins, like those present in polluted air.

Since this is not a book about diet and nutrition, it's not appropriate to delve too far into the issue here. Suffice it to say that there is an enormous amount of information available on how to incorporate exercise and a healthy diet into your lifestyle. All too often, people wait until there is something wrong—cancer or an autoimmune disease or another disabling condition—to quit smoking, change their diets, reduce stress, and take up exercise. By that time, years of abuse have left their unfortunate mark. Best to start sooner rather than later.

## REST, SLEEP, AND THE IMMUNE SYSTEM

Until a few years ago, it was a mystery why we slept—why we got tired at all. Although an eminent British physiologist, Ernest Starling, at the turn of the century described how food turned into energy, the actual process—how this translated into bodily functions—was not understood. Now we know that in order for a muscle to contract, the *chemical energy* in foods must be converted into *mechanical energy* through the complex network of the body's various systems. First, the body digests food and breaks it down into smaller components—sugars, free fatty acids, and amino acids. These are then transformed into adenosine triphosphate (ATP), which permits them to be turned into energy.

How that is accomplished depends on a long chain of events

that starts in the brain and is carried out with chemical messengers called neurotransmitters, eventually affecting either the autonomic nervous system or the endocrine (hormonal) system. The endocrine system is governed by the hypothalamus, which, as we saw earlier, is the part of the brain that is involved in the stress reaction. The hypothalamus then directs various glands to create energy for growth, metabolism, sexual activity, and physical movement. As with stress, when this transformation doesn't happen right, there's a reason. For instance, when we have a viral infection like the flu, we feel tired—which indicates pretty strongly that these systems are not working up to par and that we need to rest.

In chronic fatigue, the general listlessness and lack of energy that follow a viral infection just hang on. Interestingly, people with chronic fatigue show indications of immune dysfunction—particularly the presence of immunoglobulins in the bloodstream. Whether this has to do with the depression that follows most illnesses (depression also causes immune abnormalities) or whether there is another reason is still unknown. What it does show is that immunity and energy are linked in some way, just as immunity and stress are linked.

Today, very few people seem to get enough rest. In fact, it's become a bit of a badge of honor to talk of how little one rests, how hard one works, and how little time one has to relax. This could be a big mistake in terms of health. If your body is telling you it's tired, you should listen and figure out why. Adequate rest—together with appropriate exercise and an antioxidant-rich diet—is vital if your immune system is to keep going strong.

# Conclusion

I t's not a panacea, but MGN-3—a patented, natural food substance that's made from the outer shell of rice bran and treated and hydrolyzed under controlled conditions with enzymes from the shiitake mushroom—has been shown to increase NK-cell activity and to enhance the immune system's ability to fight cancer, AIDS, and, in all probability, viral infections such as hepatitis. It's an important discovery and worthy of major attention. Sadly, too often when people get sick they are steered toward drugs or surgery. Their own body's defenses are ignored—worse, their own immune-system defenses are reduced by the drugs and other means used to falsely eradicate disease.

We live in a hazardous world. Not in the way that it used to be—and still is in Third World countries where malaria, cholera, TB, and other diseases run rampant—but still hazardous, in that we are now exposed to many more stressors, external and internal, than we used to be. Every day, our bodies have to fend off assaults from "normal" activities, like breathing and eating. Over time, in vulnerable people, these will have an impact—which we're now seeing in the increased incidence of cancer, AIDS, chronic fatigue, hepatitis, autoimmune disorders, allergies, and asthma. The world has changed, and our views on public health measures also need to change. Globally, suggests *The Economist*, we need to focus more on "urban environmental-health problems and deal with rising rates of cancer, cardiovascular disease and mental illness."[1] We need to get with it, in other words, as a society and as individuals.

Every one of us needs to take better control of our own lives and our own health. We need to become as active in managing our own body systems as we are in our work and in our families. It's your health, your body, and nobody has the same vested interest in it as you do. Whether it's reducing stress, staying fit, eating well, or judiciously using vitamins and making other changes to our dietary habits, we need to understand our bodies and take the necessary steps to thrive—versus merely survive. But it's also important not to meekly take any and all advice that's offered. What you do and what you take should be based on evidence, science, intuition, and a host of other things. You need to figure out what's right for you. So what if someone tells you that eating carnation petals will help you avoid heart disease? Or that your only option is to take cholesterol-lowering drugs, or have radiation treatments for cancer? On what is this person—doctor, whoever it is—basing those statements? Where is the evidence? What will it mean? How will it affect your quality of life? We live in a fast-paced, consumer-driven world, where the individual has to stay alert to avoid being railroaded or taken advantage of—in health as in other matters.

As we saw in the first chapter, our immune system keeps us unique and biologically intact. Now it's up to each of us to figure out what works best for us—whether it's diet or sleep or exercise or stress. In this book, we've shown you how the immune system works and what affects it, both negatively and positively. We've also discussed what MGN-3 has been shown to do. Our hope is that some of you will find it helpful in your lives and in your path towards better health. We've given you the research data and the references. More will develop over time, as Dr. Ghoneum and his colleagues around the world continue to work on immune modulators and other substances that can enhance your natural, biological responses to disease. But in the end, it is up to you, as individuals, to stay informed, alert, and active. Nobody else can do it for you.

# Notes

## CHAPTER 1

1. Mark Lappé, *The Tao of Immunology: A Revolutionary New Understanding of Our Body's Defenses* (New York: Plenum Trade, 1997).

2. Emil R. Unanue, *Overview of the Immune System*, Vol. 1 of *Samter's Immunologic Disease*, 5th ed., ed. Michael M. Frank, et al. (Little Brown & Co., 1995), 3.

3. Lappé, *Tao of Immunology*, 44.

4. B.M. Rothschild, et al., "Geographic Distribution of Rheumatoid Arthritis in Ancient North America: Implications for Pathogenesis," *Seminars in Arthritis and Rheumatology* 22 (1992): 181–187.

5. David T. Dennis and Katherine Orloski, "Plague!" *Britannica Medical and Health Annual, 1996* (Encyclopaedia Britannica, 1996), 171–172.

6. "Health Report," *Time*, March 2, 1998, 14.

7. *The Canadian Strategy on HIV/AIDS*, HIV / AIDS Backgrounder (Ottawa: Health Canada, 1998).

8. "An ounce of prevention . . .," *The Economist*, July 4, 1998, 79.

9. Unanue, "Basic Afferent Immunology," *Overview of Immune System*, 6.

10. David Talmage, Address to the American Association of Immunology, 1988, quoted in Unanue, *Overview of Immune System.*

**Inset: Self and Not-Self: In the Beginning**

1. Lappé, *Tao of Immunology,* 96.
2. Lappé, *Tao of Immunology,* 100–101.


**CHAPTER 2**

1. "Immunity," Encyclopaedia Britannica Online, 1994–1998, www.eb.com.
2. H. Daniel Perez, "Acute Inflammation," in *Rheumatologic, Allergic and Dermatologic Disorders,* Vol. 1 of *Textbook of Internal Medicine,* 2nd ed., ed. William H. Kelley (Philadelphia: Lippincott & Co., 1992), 901.
3. "Inflammation," Britannica Online, www.eb.com.
4. "Introduction, Viruses," Britannica Online, www.eb.com.
5. "Virus," Britannica Online, www.eb.com.
6. "Drugs and Drug Action," Britannica Online, www.eb.com.
7. Lappé, *Tao of Immunology,* 104.
8. "Multiple Sclerosis," *Britannica Medical and Health Annual, 1994* (Chicago: Encyclopaedia Britannica Inc., 1994), 367.


**Inset: The Discovery of the Scavenger Cells**

1. Lappé, *Tao of Immunology,* 6.


**CHAPTER 3**

1. "Immunity," Britannica Online, www.eb.com.
2. "Jerne, Niels K.," Britannica Online, www.eb.com.

3. "The Nature of Lymphocytes," Britannica Online, www.eb.com.

4. "Poisons and Poisoning, Cellular and Humoral Immunities," Britannica Online, www.eb.com.

5. "Introduction to Clinical Immunology," in Vol. 1 of *Harrison's Principles of Internal Medicine*, 8th ed., ed. George W. Thorn, et al. (New York: McGraw-Hill Book Company, 1977), 389.

6. "Blood Cells," Britannica Online, www.eb.com.

7. "Fundamentals of Feeding Infants," *Britannica Medical and Health Annual, 1996*, 387.

8. Lappé, *Tao of Immunology*, 55.

9. Unanue, *Overview of Immune System*, 3.

10. Lappé, *Tao of Immunology*, 8.

11. "Viruses (Disease)," Britannica Online, www.eb.com.

12. "Cell-Mediated Immune Mechanisms," Britannica Online, www.eb.com.

**Inset: The Story of the Smallpox Vaccine**

1. "Edward Jenner," Britannica Online, www.eb.com.

2. "Smallpox Virus: On Death Row," *Britannica Medical and Health Annual, 1997*, 279.

**CHAPTER 4**

1. "Wright, Sir Almroth Edward," Britannica Online, www.eb.com.

2. "Antibiotic," Britannica Online, www.eb.com.

3. Editorial, *Family Practice*, Jan. 26, 1998, 8.

4. "European History and Culture, Health and Sickness," Britannica Online, www.eb.com.

5. A. J. Wakefield, et al., "Ileal-Lymphoid-Modular Hyperplasia,

Non-specific Colitis, and Pervasive Developmental Disorder in Children," *The Lancet* 351 (Feb. 28, 1998): 637–641.

6. Lappé, *Tao of Immunology*, 252.
7. Lappé, *Tao of Immunology*, 254.
8. "Vaccines," *Pharmaguide*, (Merck Frosst Canada Inc., 1998).
9. "An ounce of prevention," *The Economist*, July 4, 1998, 79.

**CHAPTER 5**

1. Lappé, *Tao of Immunology*, 36–37.

**CHAPTER 6**

1. "Immune Deficiencies," Britannica Online, www.eb.com.
2. "What Is an Allergic Reaction?", Web site for patients made available through the American Academy of Allergy Asthma and Immunology, accessible through Britannica Online or directly at www.aaaai.org.
3. "Asthma (Update)," *Britannica Medical and Health Annual 1995*, 234.
4. *Health*, May/June 1998, 20.
5. Lappé, *Tao of Immunology*, 243.
6. P.G. Burney, et al., "Has the Prevalence of Asthma Increased in Children? Evidence from the National Study of Health and Growth, Department of Public Health Medicine," *British Medical Journal* 300 (June 23, 1990): 1652–1653.
7. Lappé, *Tao of Immunology*, 244.
8. S. O. Shaheen, et al., "Measles and Atopy in Guinea-Bissau," *The Lancet* 347 (June 1996): 1792–1796.
9. S. O. Shaheen, et al., "Cell-mediated Immunity after Measles in Guinea-Bissau," *British Medical Journal* 313 (Oct. 1996): 969–974.
10. P. Aaby, et al., "No Persistent T-lymphocyte Immunosuppression or Increased Mortality after Measles Infection: A Commu-

nity Study from Guinea-Bissau," *Pediatric Infectious Disease Journal* 15 (Jan. 1996): 39–44.

## CHAPTER 7

1. Lappé, *Tao of Immunology*, 238.
2. "Autoimmunity," Britannica Online, www.eb.com.
3. Mark Lappé, *Evolutionary Medicine* (San Francisco: Sierra Club Books, 1995), Chapter 12.
4. C.M. Black, "Overview of Systemic Sclerosis," *The Lancet* 347 (1996): 1453–1458.
5. Lappé, *Tao of Immunology*, 122.
6. "Lupus," *Canadian Medical Association Encyclopaedia*, Vol. 2, 654.
7. "Immunity," Britannica Online, www.eb.com.
8. Lappé, *Tao of Immunology*, 124.
9. Lappé, *Tao of Immunology*, 116.

### Inset: MHC and Tissue Transplantation

1. Unanue, *Overview of Immune System*, 7.
2. R.E. Billington, et al., "Actively Acquired Tolerance of Foreign Cells," *Nature* 172 (1953): 603, quoted in Unanue, *Overview of Immune System*, 6.

## CHAPTER 8

1. Laurence Cherry, "On the Real Benefits of Eustress: An Interview with Dr. Hans Selye," *Psychology Today*, March 1978, 60.
2. Lappé, *Tao of Immunology*, 132.
3. Lappé, *Tao of Immunology*, 133.
4. Henry Dreher, *The Immune Power Personality* (New York: Penguin, 1995), 23.

5. W.T. Boyce, et al., "Psychobiologic Reactivity to Stress and Childhood Respiratory Illnesses: Results of Two Prospective Studies," *Psychosomatic Medicine* 57 (1995): 411–422.

6. Dreher, *Immune Power Personality*, 26.

7. Lappé, *Tao of Immunology*, 136.

8. Mamdooh Ghoneum, "Susceptibility of Natural Killer Cell Activity of Old Rats to Stress," *Immunology* 60 (1987): 461–465.

9. *Health*, April 1998, 15.

10. A. Gershon Ballin, et al., "The Antidepressant Fluvoxamine Increases Natural Killer Cell Counts in Cancer Patients," *Israeli Journal of Medical Sciences* 33 (Nov. 1997):720–723.

11. Dreher, *Immune Power Personality*, 22–23.

12. J. Itami, et al., "Laughter and Immunity," *Shinshin-Igaku* 34 (1994): 565–571.

13. Lappé, *Tao of Immunology*, 143.

14. Katherine Griffin, "Karashi in America?" *InHealth*, May/June 1991, 43.

15. "Medical Quotes," *Journal of the History of Medicine and Allied Sciences* 13 (1958): 42.

16. "UN Seeks to Outlaw DDT, Other Toxins," syndicated article from *Washington Post, Vancouver Sun*, June 29, 1998.

17. Aristo Vojdani, et al., "Immune Alteration Associated with Exposure to Toxic Chemicals," *Toxicology and Industrial Health*, 8 (1992): 239.

**CHAPTER 9**

1. "How AIDS Began," *The Economist*, February 7, 1998, 81.

2. "Numbers," *Time*, July 13, 1998, 12.

3. "AIDS Update," *Britannica Medical and Health Annual*, 1997, 164.

4. Lappé, *Tao of Immunology*, 221.

5. Lappé, *Tao of Immunology*, 222.

6. "HIV and AIDS," *Pharmaguide* (Merck Frosst Canada), 2.

7. "AIDS Update," *Britannica Medical and Health Annual 1997*, 165.

8. Lappé, *Tao of Immunology*, 226.

9. Glenn Wanamaker, "Successfully Containing HIV," *Family Practice*, June 15, 1998, 26.

10. "An Ounce of Prevention," *The Economist*, July 4, 1998, 79.

**CHAPTER 10**

1. James MacGowan, "Cancer: The Disease of Civilization?" *Family Practice*, Feb. 19, 1996, 47.

2. *University of California Wellness Letter*, Aug. 1998, 8.

3. Sheryl L. Parker, et al., "Cancer Statistics, 1996," *CA:A Cancer Journal for Clinicians* 65 (Jan/Feb 1996): 5–27.

4. Pippa Wysong, "Canadian Cancer Statistics—1998 Report," *The Medical Post*, April 21, 1998, 2.

5. Sallie Tisdale, *The Sorcerer's Apprentice: Medical Miracles and Other Disasters* (New York: Henry Holt, 1988), 183.

6. A. Vojdani, et al., "Minimizing Cancer Risk Using Molecular Techniques: A Review," *Toxicology and Industrial Health* 13 (1997): 589–626.

7. I. William Lane and Linda Comac, *Sharks Don't Get Cancer* (New York: Avery Publishing Group, 1992).

8. I. William Lane and Linda Comac, *Sharks Still Don't Get Cancer* (New York: Avery Publishing Group, 1996).

9. "Immunity against Cancer," Britannica Online, www.eb.com.

10. Lappé, *Tao of Immunology*, 183.

11. Lappé, *Tao of Immunology*, 162.

12. Mamdooh Ghoneum, et al., "Change in Tumour Cell-Lymphocyte Interactions with Age," *Hematological Oncology* 8 (1990): 71–80.

13. Mamdooh Ghoneum, et al., "Immunomodulatory and anti-cancer effects of active hemicellulose compound," *International Journal of Immunotherapy* 9 (1995): 23–28.

## CHAPTER 11

1. T. Timonen, "Natural Killer Cells: Endothelial Interactions, Migration and Target Cell Recognition," *Journal of Leukocyte Biology* 62 (Dec. 1997): 699–701.
2. F. Komatsu and K. Kihara, "Natural Killer (NK) and Lymphokine-Activated Killer (LAK) Activities in a Patient Who Recovered from Cancer, and the Characteristics of LAK Cells Generated from CD4-, CD8-, and CD8+ Peripheral Blood Lymphocytes," *Clinical Immunology and Immunopathology* 77 (Oct. 1995): 75–81.
3. A. Esp'i, et al., "Relationship of Curative Surgery on Natural Killer Cell Activity in Colorectal Cancer," *Diseases of the Colon and Rectum* 39 (April 1996): 429–434.
4. S.M. Levy, et al., "Immunologic and Psychosocial Predictors of Disease Recurrence in Patients with Early Stage Breast Cancer," *Behavioral Medicine* 17 (Summer 1991): 67–75.
5. J. Brittenden, et al., "Natural Killer Cells and Cancer," *Cancer* 77 (April 1, 1996): 1226–1243.
6. Bernie Siegel, *Peace, Love & Healing* (New York: Harper and Row, 1989), 130–131.
7. Mamdooh Ghoneum, et al., "Immunomodulatory and Anti-cancer Effects of Active Hemicellulose Compound," *Journal of Immunotherapy* 11 (1995): 23–28.
8. Mamdooh Ghoneum, et al., "MGN-3 as Conjunctive Therapy in Multiple Myeloma—Role of Activated Natural Killer Cells (Case Report), Japan Functional Food Research Association Web site, health-station.com.
9. Mamdooh Ghoneum, et al., "Modulation of Natural Killer Cell Activity as a Possible Conjunctive Method in Treatment of

Ovarian Carcinoma Utilizing MGN-3, a Modified Zylose from Rice Bran," Japan Functional Food Research Association Web site, health-station.com

10. Mamdooh Ghoneum, et al., "Anti-HIV Activity *in Vitro* of MGN-3, an Activated Arabinoxylane from Rice Bran," Japan Functional Food Research Association Web site, health-station.com.

**CHAPTER 12**

1. Lappé, *Tao of Immunology*, 147.
2. "Great Going," *Health*, April 1998, 34.
3. Lappé, *Tao of Immunology*, 146.
4. "Can Antioxidants Save Your Life?" *University of California Wellness Letter*, July 1998, 4.

**CONCLUSION**

1. "Repositioning the WHO," *The Economist*, May 9, 1998, 79.

# Glossary

*Italicized words* are defined elsewhere in the glossary.

**acquired immunity.** Any form of *immunity* that is acquired after birth. A naturally acquired immunity occurs as a result of an individual's having a disease. An artificially acquired immunity is a response to vaccination.

**acute-phase reaction.** The *immune system's* most basic first step in defense of the body. During this reaction, *microphages* and *macrophages* surround and digest *bacteria* and other foreign particles in the blood.

**adrenaline.** A stress hormone produced by the adrenal gland that stimulates the sympathetic nervous system and is instrumental in attention and memory.

**allergen.** An ordinarily harmless substance that provokes an allergic response in a sensitive individual. Common allergens include animal dander, pollen, certain drugs, lint, *bacteria*, and some foods.

**allergic reaction.** An *immune system* response to an *allergen*. Common allergic reactions include sneezing, runny eyes, and hives. This type of reaction is also called immediate hypersensitivity.

**allergy.** An inappropriate response by the *immune system* to contact with a normally harmless substance called an *allergen*.

**allostatic systems.** The parts of the nervous system that control heartbeat, blood pressure, and hormonal responses, as well as the cardiovascular, metabolic, and *immune systems*.

**anaphylaxis.** A severe, potentially life-threatening allergic response to a foreign substance (*antigen*) with which an individual has had previous contact. Responses can include skin redness and swelling, itching, and water build-up. In severe cases, there may be extremely low blood pressure, spasm of the lungs, and shock.

**angiogenesis.** See *neovascularization*.

**antibiotic.** A substance capable of killing or inhibiting the growth of microorganisms, especially *bacteria*.

**antibody.** A protein that is created by the *immune system* in response to the presence of a foreign organism or toxin, and is capable of destroying or neutralizing the invader. Each antibody reacts to a specific foreign body, or *antigen*.

**antigen.** A foreign substance that stimulates the production of an *antibody*.

**antihistamine.** A substance that blocks the action of *histamines*.

**apoptosis.** Cell death that occurs naturally, as opposed to cell death from disease or injury. Apoptosis can be caused by various external stimuli, such as high heat, bacterial toxins, chemotherapy, certain toxic chemicals, and ultraviolet light.

**Arabinoxylan Compound (MGN-3).** A patented blend of rice-bran *hemicellulose* B and shiitake mushroom. This compound dramatically increases the activity of *natural killer (NK) cells*, and may be useful in fighting cancer.

**autoimmune disorder.** Any condition in which the *immune system* attacks the body's own tissues, causing damage and interfering with normal functioning.

**bacteria.** Single-celled microorganisms. Some bacteria can cause disease. Other bacteria—the so-called "friendly" bacteria—are normally present in the body and perform such useful functions as aiding digestion and protecting the body from harmful invading organisms.

**bacteriophage.** Any *virus* that causes *bacteria* to disintegrate. Bacteriophages are also referred to as phages.

**B cell.** A type of *lymphocyte* that searches out foreign invaders, and, in response, stimulates the formation of *immunoglobulins*.

**biological response modifier (BRM).** A nontoxic substance that has a measurable effect on biological responses, such as those of the *immune system*.

**cell-mediated immunity.** Refers to the growth of *T cells* after exposure to a foreign substance (*antigen*). The T cells go to work each time they meet the same substance. Cell-mediated immunity, which is also called cellular immunity, helps the body resist infection caused by *viruses* and some *bacteria*, and also plays a role in delayed allergic responses.

**cellular immunity.** See *cell-mediated immunity*.

**CTL-induced lysis.** See *cytotoxic T lymphocyte*.

**cytokines.** Proteins that acts as important regulators of the *immune system*.

**cytotoxic.** Damaging to cells.

**cytotoxic T lymphocyte.** A type of *lymphocyte* that recognizes foreign *antigens* on the surface of a cancer cell or other target cells, binds to the antigens, and destroys the target cell by injecting it with destructive chemicals in a process called CTL-induced lysis.

**DNA (deoxyribonucleic acid).** The substance in the cell nucleus that contains the cell's genetic blueprint and determines the type of life form into which a cell will develop.

**free radical.** An atom, molecule, or fragment of a molecule that has at least one unpaired electron, making it highly unstable and ready to react with other atoms or molecules. Free radicals can attack and damage cells, contributing to aging and disease.

**granulocyte.** A microphage that contains a granule or grain. A granulocyte is a type of scavenger cell.

**hapten.** An *antigen* that does not provoke an immune response.

**hemicellulose.** A kind of dietary fiber that is useful in aiding gastric functions and promoting the growth of beneficial intestinal *bacteria.*

**histamine.** A chemical produced by the immune system in response to contact with an *allergen.* Histamines cause bronchial tube muscles to constrict, small blood vessels to dilate, and secretions from mucous membranes to increase, all of which result in the sneezing, itching, and discomfort of an *allergic reaction.*

**histocompatability.** The ability to accept transplants of tissues from one individual to another. Histocompatability depends on identical genetic constitution of both individuals.

**humoral immunity.** A condition that results from the development and continuing presence of circulating *antibodies* that are produced by the body's defense system. When the antibodies encounter their specific *antigens,* they either damage the invasive cells or alert the white blood cells to attack.

**hypersusceptibility.** The predisposition of an individual to react to a specific chemical.

**idiosyncrasy.** A genetic predisposition of an individual to react to a specific chemical; in other words, *hypersusceptibility* that is genetically determined.

**immediate hypersensitivity.** See *allergic reaction.*

**immune system.** A complex system of organs, tissues, cells, and proteins whose chief function is to identify and eliminate invaders, such as harmful *bacteria.* The liver, spleen, thymus, bone marrow, and lymphatic system all play vital roles in the proper functioning of the immune system.

**immunity.** The condition of being able to resist and overcome disease or *infection.*

**immunocompetence.** The ability to produce *antibodies* or *cell-mediated immunity* when exposed to a foreign substance (*antigen*).

**immunodeficiency.** A defect in the functioning of the *immune system* that can be inherited or acquired, reversible or permanent.

Immunodeficiency renders the body more susceptible to illness of every type, especially infectious illnesses.

**immunogen.** Any substance able to provoke an immune response or cause *immunity.*

**immunoglobulin.** A protein molecule functioning as a specific *antibody.*

**immunotherapy.** The treatment of disease by using techniques intended to stimulate or strengthen the *immune system.*

**infection.** An invasion of the body by organisms such as *viruses,* harmful *bacteria,* or fungi that results in disease.

**infectious disease.** A disease that is set in motion by the presence of minute microorganisms, usually *bacteria,* and is capable of being transmitted or of causing *infection.*

**inflammation.** A reaction to illness or injury characterized by swelling, warmth, and redness.

**interferon.** A protein that is produced by the *immune system* in response to the presence of a *virus,* and can prevent the virus from reproducing or infecting other cells.

**interleukin-1 (IL-1).** A protein of the *immune system* that activates resting *T cells* and *macrophage* cells, enhancing the immune response and assisting in the repair of damage.

**killer (K) cell.** A type of cell that is similar to a *natural killer (NK) cell,* but destroys foreign substances through a different mechanism. K cells help certain *B cells* to kill *viruses* by injecting a toxic substance into the virus, and thereby causing it to self-destruct. K cells are also called lymphokine-activated killer (LAK) cells.

**Koch phenomenon.** An immune-mediated reaction to a microorganism in which the immune response does more harm than that done by the microorganism itself, and may even lead to death.

**leukocyte.** Any white blood cell that helps protect the body from *infection* and disease.

**lymphocyte.** A type of small white blood cell that is responsible for the development of specific *immunities*. Lymphocytes are found in lymph, blood, and other specialized tissues, such as the bone marrow and tonsils. *B cells, T cells,* and *cytotoxic T lymphocytes* are considered lymphocytes. Natural killer (NK) cells are considered a special subset of lymphocytes.

**lymphokine.** Any of a group of substances produced by the cells of the immune system when exposed to foreign substances (*antigens*). Lymphokines are not *antibodies*, but rather perform such functions as stimulating the production of *lymphocytes* and activating other immune cells.

**lymphokine-activated killer (LAK) cell.** See *killer (K) cell.*

**macrophage.** A large cell that can surround and digest foreign substances in the body, such as *bacteria.* Also called scavenger cells, macrophages are found throughout the body, with the greatest number being found in the spleen.

**major histocompatability complex (MHC).** A group of proteins on the cell membrane that help distinguish between the cell's own molecules and invading molecules.

**mast cell.** A connective tissue cell whose activation causes a variety of reactions, of which muscle constriction is the most common. Mast cells also cause relaxation of blood vessels in the skin or in the whole body, which can lead to *anaphylaxis.*

**MGN-3.** See *Arabinoxylan Compound.*

**microphage.** A small cell able to take in and digest small particles, such as *bacteria.* Also called scavenger cells, microphages come in two forms: *leukocytes* and *granulocytes.*

**mitosis.** The process by which the body makes new cells for both growth and repair of injured tissue.

**natural killer (NK) cell.** A cell that is able to bind to cancer cells and, to a lesser extent, to *viruses,* and destroy them through the use of granules, which the NK cell uses much as a gun uses bullets.

**necrosis.** Local tissue death that occurs in groups of cells because of disease or injury.

**neovascularization.** The development of new blood vessels. Also called angiogenesis, neovascularization is a common feature of cancerous tissue.

**neuropeptide.** A chemical that seems to act as a messenger between the brain and the *immune system*.

**neutrophil.** A circulating white blood cell that acts to ingest and destroy *bacteria*, cell debris, and solid particles in the blood.

**nonspecific immunity.** A general response of the *immune system* in which cells such as *microphages* search for invaders such as *bacteria*. This contrasts with specific immunity, in which the body reacts to specific invading microorganisms.

**Pasteurella pestis.** See *plague*.

**pasteurization.** The process of destroying or retarding the growth of microorganisms in milk and other foods by heating the food to a specific temperature for a specific period of time.

**pathogen.** A disease-causing toxin or microorganism.

**phage.** See *bacteriophage*.

**phagocytosis.** A process in which a substance is engulfed and then held or digested by a cell.

**plague.** Formerly used to describe any epidemic causing great mortality, this term now refers to a specific infectious disease caused by the bacillus *Pasteurella pestis*.

**prostaglandin.** Any of a number of hormonelike chemicals that are made in the body from essential fatty acids, and have important effects on body functions. Prostaglandins influence the secretion of hormones and enzymes, and help regulate the inflammatory response, blood pressure, and blood clotting time.

**psychoneuroimmunology (PNI).** A new field of study that looks at the mind-body interaction and its effects on disease.

**retrovirus.** A type of *virus* that can convert *RNA* into *DNA*, and thereby use genetic material to make the protein it needs to survive. HIV is an example of a retrovirus.

**RNA (ribonucleic acid).** A complex protein found in plant and animal cells, as well as viruses, that carries coded genetic information from the DNA, in the cell nucleus, to protein-producing cell structures called ribosomes.

**scavenger cell.** See *macrophage; microphage.*

**sterilization.** A technique for destroying microorganisms through the use of heat, water, chemicals, or gases.

**stress.** The body's nonspecific response to any demand placed upon it, whether physical or psychological. When excessive and prolonged, stress can lead to disease.

**stressor.** Anything that causes *stress* by taxing the body's physical or mental resources.

**synergy.** An interaction between two or more substances in which the substances' action together is greater than the sum of their individual actions.

**T cell.** A type of *lymphocyte* that plays a major role in *cell-mediated immunity.* T cells are involved in the direct attack against invading organisms.

**virus.** Any of a large class of minute parasitic organic structures that are capable of infecting plants and animals by reproducing within their cells. Because they cannot reproduce outside of a host organism's cells, viruses are not technically considered living organisms.

# Index

# Healthy Habits
### *are easy to come by—*
## IF YOU KNOW WHERE TO LOOK!

### Get the latest information on:
- **better health • diet & weight loss**
- **the latest nutritional supplements**
- **herbal healing • homeopathy and more**

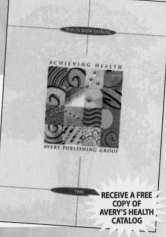

RECEIVE A FREE
COPY OF
AVERY'S HEALTH
CATALOG

## COMPLETE AND RETURN THIS CARD RIGHT AWAY!

**Where did you purchase this book?**
- ❑ bookstore
- ❑ supermarket
- ❑ health food store
- ❑ other (please specify)_____
- ❑ pharmacy

Name_____

Street Address_____

City_____State_____Zip_____

---

## GIVE ONE TO A FRIEND ...

# Healthy Habits
### *are easy to come by—*
## IF YOU KNOW WHERE TO LOOK!

### Get the latest information on:
- **better health • diet & weight loss**
- **the latest nutritional supplements**
- **herbal healing • homeopathy and more**

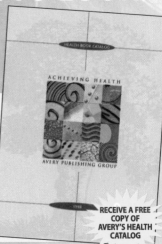

RECEIVE A FREE
COPY OF
AVERY'S HEALTH
CATALOG

## COMPLETE AND RETURN THIS CARD RIGHT AWAY!

**Where did you purchase this book?**
- ❑ bookstore
- ❑ supermarket
- ❑ health food store
- ❑ other (please specify)_____
- ❑ pharmacy

Name_____

Street Address_____

City_____State_____Zip_____

# Avery Publishing Group

**120 Old Broadway**
**Garden City Park, NY 11040**

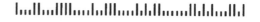

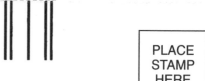

# Avery Publishing Group

**120 Old Broadway**
**Garden City Park, NY 11040**